Children of AIDS

Children of AIDS
Africa's Orphan Crisis

Emma Guest

Pluto Press
LONDON • STERLING, VIRGINIA

UNIVERSITY OF NATAL PRESS
Pietermaritzburg
South Africa

First published 2001 by Pluto Press
345 Archway Road, London N6 5AA
and 22883 Quicksilver Drive,
Sterling, VA 20166–2012, USA

www.plutobooks.com

Published in South Africa by
University of Natal Press
Private Bag X01
Scottsville 3209
South Africa
E-mail: books@nu.ac.za

British Library Cataloguing in Publication Data
A catalogue record for this book is available from the British Library

Library of Congress Cataloging in Publication Data
Guest, Emma, 1970–
   Children of AIDS : Africa's orphan crisis / Emma Guest.
     p. cm.
Includes index.
  ISBN 0 7453 1769 3
   1. Orphans—Services for—Africa. 2. Children of AIDS
patients—Services for—Africa. 3. AIDS (Disease)—Social
aspects—Africa. I. Title.
  HV1337 .G84 2001
  362.73'096—dc21

                              00–012928

ISBN 0 7453 1769 3 hardback (Pluto)
ISBN 0 86980 992 X (Southern Africa only)

10 09 08 07 06 05 04 03 02 01
10 9 8 7 6 5 4 3 2 1

Designed and produced for the publishers by
Chase Publishing Services, Sidmouth, EX10 9QG
Typeset from disk by Stanford DTP Services, Northampton
Printed in the European Union by TJ International, Padstow, England

For Robert and Heidi

Contents

Preface

Deadlier than war, deadlier than tyranny, deadlier even than malaria, AIDS is silently tearing Africa apart. The epidemic is throwing millions of households into turmoil. Often the middle generation is wiped out, and children and the elderly are left to fend for themselves.

In this book, I have tried to give a glimpse of the lives of a few of these survivors, whether struggling to keep their families intact or eking out a precarious existence on the streets. And I have tried to recount the tribulations of those who try to help this new generation of orphans, often despite minimal resources and obstructive bureaucracy. It is the story of people's lives after AIDS.

'A book on AIDS orphans? How depressing!' This was the reaction of almost everyone I met in South Africa. Friends were bemused. Why would anyone choose to spend 18 months researching and writing a book on such a gloomy subject?

I am a white foreigner in Africa. This status bestows numerous obstacles but also a few freedoms. As an outsider, it was not always easy to gain people's trust. But I could bring a fresh perspective to the subject. Many of the courageous people I met during the course of my research – social workers, doctors, volunteers – devoted all their time and effort to keeping their various projects afloat. Finding enough food to keep orphans in their care healthy, ferrying sick children down awful roads to distant clinics, scrabbling for funds ... with so many immediate and pressing concerns, one could hardly expect them to spend much time studying the experiences of other people in similar situations in other parts of the continent.

I felt that such a study would prove useful. So I interviewed dozens of people at the front line, if I can call it that, of the battle against AIDS. In these conversations, I tried to find out three things. How does AIDS affect African families? How do Africans cope with the epidemic? And what can others do to help?

I pursued my research in three very different countries: Uganda, Zambia and South Africa.

I chose Uganda because the AIDS epidemic there is mature. HIV prevalence has peaked, albeit at a horrifyingly high level, and is now falling. Uganda is poor, but its government is open and has shown an impressive commitment to fighting the disease. Posters everywhere warn about the virus. President Yoweri Museveni urges abstinence or safe sex in almost every speech. A multitude of non-governmental organisations (NGOs) is given free rein to preach prevention in any way they choose.

Zambia is enjoying less success. Roughly 20 per cent of Zambian adults are infected.[1] The country has perhaps the second highest proportion of orphans in the world (after Rwanda) with an estimated 27 per cent of children under 15 having lost their mother, father or both parents by 2000, mainly to AIDS.[2] Tackling AIDS in Zambia is made harder by the fact that the country is poor and the government is somewhat ineffectual and sometimes corrupt.

Finally, I chose South Africa because it is the richest and most developed country in the region, but still has problems curbing the epidemic. AIDS came late to South Africa, partly because the place was so isolated during apartheid. People in the Western Cape, the southernmost province, still talk of a 'window of opportunity' to learn from other provinces, and the country's northern neighbours, where the epidemic is already severe. But this window is closing fast. South Africa now has over 4 million infected citizens, more than any other country.[3] The South African government woke up to the crisis at the end of 1998, but is still floundering. The president, Thabo Mbeki, has flirted with discredited theories about the cause of the disease. Meanwhile, 1,700 South Africans contract HIV every day.

Little in my previous experience prepared me for this task. I came from a comfortable British background, the daughter of a country doctor and a marriage guidance counsellor. Before I came to Africa, I did a job I loved: publicising a charity called The Samaritans, a helpline for the suicidal that was established by an eccentric vicar in 1953. My days were spent encouraging sometimes cynical journalists to write sympathetically about depression and suicide.

Outside work, I took an interest in AIDS. Once a week, I'd meet up with a woman living with the disease. We'd sit in a pub if she was feeling good, or a hospital if she wasn't, and I'd listen to whatever she wanted to talk about. It never felt like a chore.

She was a survivor. Originally from Kenya, she made her living importing African artwork and selling it from a stall in a London market. Britain's National Health Service provided her with anti-retroviral drugs – dozens of pills a day – to keep the virus at bay. The drugs work, but they have nasty side effects, so my buddy[4] refused to swallow them. She'd collect her prescription, to keep the doctors from nagging, but then stockpile the bottles in her bedroom.

The irony of all this struck me when I came to Africa. On the world's poorest and most AIDS-ravaged continent, AIDS drugs are impossibly expensive. The pills that my buddy received for free, but discarded, cost about $10,000 a year. In a typical African country, providing them to everyone with HIV would cost more than the entire national income, leaving nothing over for food or clothes. Activists lobby for cheaper medicines, but even at huge discounts, probably only South Africa will be able to afford even a limited number of the treatments available in the West.

I came to Africa by chance. I met my future husband at a wedding and three months later we were engaged. Then his employer, the *Economist* magazine, asked him to go to South Africa. I agreed to accompany him. After seven years working in London, I was ready for a change. We got married, waved goodbye to everything familiar and flew to Johannesburg the next day.

I knew very little about what I was going to. I'd heard that AIDS was a big problem in Africa, but had no idea of the level of suffering it was causing. I'd also naively assumed that there'd be plenty I could do to help. But I swiftly learnt that there are few spaces for full-time public relations staff in South Africa's small and impecunious NGOs. The fact that I was white and foreign did not help either. Four years after apartheid, my background aroused distrust.

So I freelanced. I provided consulting services about AIDS to companies, and ghost-wrote reports on the subject for independent consultants, who in turn had been contracted to supply them to the government or NGOs.

While researching my various reports, I noticed that there wasn't a book on AIDS orphans in Africa. The disease was, at last, featured daily in the South African press and on television. But little thought was being devoted to the estimated 2–4.5 million AIDS orphans South Africa would be home to by 2010.[5]

It is perhaps presumptuous on my part to write a book about AIDS in Africa. It is a controversial field, riven with passionate disputes and hair-trigger sensitivities. 'What are your credentials?' I have sometimes been asked, and, 'What's your methodology?'

This book is unapologetically anecdotal. It is the result of gently questioning people about their lives and faithfully transcribing their words. By recording their stories, I hope to shed light on different aspects of, and responses to, the AIDS orphan crisis.

To persuade people to open up to me, I had to overcome linguistic, cultural and racial obstacles. I would usually start by contacting local NGOs. Once I had gained their trust, I would be introduced to people who'd benefited from their services and the NGO staff would sometimes translate local languages for me. Consequently, many of the individuals featured in this book are relatively lucky. They had at least found lifelines. Some had also been selected, by the NGO that looked after them, for being 'success stories'. Most African families receive no outside assistance, so AIDS orphans beyond the reach of NGOs and researchers are likely to be much worse off.

In Zambia and Uganda, it is assumed that a *muzungu* (white) visiting a project represents a donor agency. Children and grandmothers would constantly ask me for money. My response that I was there not with cash, but with a pen, was often greeted with incomprehension. Of what possible use was my book to this particular street child? He wanted shoes now.

Everywhere I went, I observed that projects tend to run on the energy and ideas of a single individual. If that person leaves, they often collapse. These caring individuals get things done, but not always in a focused, strategic way. Relationships with the civil servants and foreign donors who approve their funding are sometimes fraught. NGO leaders, believing so passionately in their cause, sometimes find it hard to learn from, or co-operate with, others who have different ideas about how to reach the same goals. During one AIDS conference in South Africa in 1999, when the discussions reached an impasse, a priest who runs an orphanage leapt up, crying, 'There are kids dying out there!'

No one working in the field, who sees death daily, can figure out why everyone else doesn't share their sense of panic. The projections for the numbers of AIDS orphans are terrifying. Without help, many of these children will end up uneducated, alienated and on the streets.

And yet some African governments seem to lack a sense of urgency about the crisis. In places where corruption is widespread and politics simply the easiest way to get rich, government funds are often squandered rather than used to alleviate poverty. The naked self-interest of some of the politicians I met shocked me.

How would rich countries respond to a similar crisis? Perhaps the question is futile. In Western Europe, Japan and North America the basic needs of the poorest – enough to eat, a roof and a pair of trainers – are largely taken care of. Governments in rich countries have the time and money to concern themselves with the psychosocial impact of their much smaller AIDS epidemics.

In the US, where there were about 80,000 AIDS orphans in 2000, there are armies of counsellors to help children with their 'grief work'.[6] Children are encouraged to talk through their feelings of denial, abandonment, anger and sadness, in peer support groups, family therapy or one-to-one sessions. Dying parents make 'memory' videos.

Before coming to South Africa, I had been working for an organisation which believed that everyone had the right to be listened to, and that an individual's emotional wellbeing depended upon such an outlet. I swiftly learnt that before you can worry about a child's mental state, you have to make sure she has something to eat, and maybe some antibiotics.

The lives of many AIDS orphans are bleak, but I hope that readers will not find this book wholly depressing. It's full of stories of extraordinary resilience. Of course, many of my subjects have little choice but to be resilient, but their struggles are still frequently awe-inspiring. The orphans, aunts and grandmothers I've interviewed battle on despite poverty and bereavement. When I meet a 17-year-old who is bringing up her siblings alone, I'm humbled.

I hope, too, that the example of the social workers, NGO staff and international donors I have described will inspire others to get involved or give money to a reputable charity. Details of the organisations featured in this book can be found at the end.

I am grateful for the expert input of Professor Alan Whiteside, Dr Neil McKerrow, Professor Brian Williams and Lynn van Lith.

Finally, I would like to thank all those who have let me into their lives. I have changed names where necessary to protect people's privacy. But all the stories, sometimes unfortunately, sometimes happily, are true.

Introduction

A 13-year-old Kenyan AIDS orphan gave away her virginity in exchange for an apple. Asked why, she replied, 'No one's ever given me anything before.'[1]

The tragedy of AIDS does not end with the death of the sufferer. It continues through the lives of the children who are orphaned. In Africa, where the epidemic is at its worst, a whole generation of children is growing up without parents.

Just how bad is the AIDS epidemic? No one knows for sure. The Joint United Nations Programme on HIV/AIDS (UNAIDS) estimates that, at the end of the twentieth century, nearly 19 million people had died of AIDS around the world, leaving over 13 million orphans.[2]

Africa has been struck the hardest. About 70 per cent of the world's 34 million HIV-positive people live south of the Sahara desert and about 95 per cent of the world's AIDS orphans are African. In seven countries, an extraordinary one in five adults (defined as those aged 15 to 49) are thought to be infected. They're all in southern Africa. In the worst hit country, Botswana, over a third of adults are infected. In 1998, South Africa had an adult HIV prevalence of about 13 per cent. By 2000, 20 per cent were infected. That's over four million infected people, the largest number in any country. Unless sexual behaviour changes, between six and ten million South Africans, from a population of about 42 million, may die of AIDS in the next 10–15 years.[3]

The figures are staggering, perhaps 19 million dead already and 13 million grieving children around the world. With 34 million currently infected and likely to die during the next decade, many more children face being orphaned. The United States Agency for International Development (USAID) estimates that 44 million children under 15, in 34 developing countries, will have lost one or both parents by 2010, mostly to AIDS.[4]

But how reliable are these statistics? Some African countries gather virtually no information about HIV/AIDS. Others extrapolate national statistics from pockets of data, usually surveys of the HIV prevalence amongst pregnant women attending antenatal clinics.

Only UNAIDS attempts to track and compare the epidemic in different countries. It's a difficult job when there are no exact counts of births and deaths, let alone HIV and AIDS cases, in Africa. Few HIV/AIDS cases are actually diagnosed and because of the stigma surrounding the disease, doctors rarely put AIDS as the cause of death on patients' death certificates. Instead they say the patient died of tuberculosis or pneumonia, keeping silent about the virus that destroyed his immune system and allowed these opportunistic infections to kill him. Such tact saves families from extra pain but obscures the truth. African HIV/AIDS data will always be approximate, but UNAIDS's regular reports offer a useful *impression* of the scale and trends of the epidemic on a continent where the vast majority of HIV-positive people don't know they're infected.

African AIDS orphan statistics are even muddier because they're calculated using even more assumptions (such as average numbers of children per mother, allowing for a reduction in fertility and increase in infant deaths caused by HIV) and because definitions vary of what an orphan is. Some statisticians include children who have lost their mother or both parents. Others include children who have lost either or both parents, or just those who have lost both.

However rough the statistics are, it's clear that the HIV/AIDS epidemic could be as catastrophic for Africa as the Black Death was for mediaeval Europe. In fact, it could be worse. Bubonic plague wiped out roughly a third of Europe's population within 15 years in the fourteenth century. Those who survived, however, grew less poor because there was suddenly a shortage of hands to plough the fields, so wages rose. Africa, after AIDS, is unlikely to enjoy even this scrap of comfort, because unemployment and under-employment are so widespread.

Why has Africa been worse affected than anywhere else? It's widely accepted that AIDS began in Africa, so the virus didn't have far to travel. Other important factors include poverty, patterns of sexual networking, cultural practices, the subordinate position of women, wars and migrant labour. Most African governments' efforts to curb AIDS have been ineffectual or non-existent.

The human immuno-deficiency virus probably originated in western central Africa in the 1920s or 1930s. HIV-1 is known to be a strain of a virus that had existed for many years in chimpanzees, without harming them. Another rarer strain, HIV-2, came from sooty mangabey monkeys. The virus probably crossed from apes to humans when the two species' blood intermingled, perhaps when someone with a cut on her hand was preparing chimp meat for the pot. It was only identified 50 years later.

Other theories about the origin of AIDS abound, some more serious than others. Journalist Edward Hooper, in his book *The River*, argued that doctors inadvertently sparked off the epidemic with contaminated polio vaccines in the Belgian Congo in the 1950s.[5]

A small group of scientists, known as the 'AIDS dissidents' (nicknamed 'Flat-earthers' by some) believe that HIV is not the cause of AIDS. In the developed world, they attribute the disease to recreational drug use, promiscuity and even the drugs prescribed to combat AIDS. They blame the epidemic in Africa on malnutrition, parasitic infection and poor sanitation. Some don't believe that HIV/AIDS is infectious. Others don't believe AIDS exists.

Conspiracy theorist and Ku Klux Klan supporter, William Cooper believes that the *Illuminati* (an alleged secret society of powerful scientists, politicians, bankers and so on) deliberately manufactured AIDS in order to wipe out homosexuals, blacks and Hispanics.[6] Mr Cooper claims that HIV was introduced to Africa via the smallpox vaccine in 1977. He also has some outlandish ideas about space aliens and the assassination of John F. Kennedy.

Such theories wouldn't be worth mentioning if they didn't have a dangerous allure. Some intelligent people believe that the HIV virus was concocted in a western laboratory with the intention of killing off Africans. Perhaps unsurprisingly, given the atrocities of colonial and apartheid regimes, paranoia lingers.

South African President Thabo Mbeki sought advice from American 'AIDS dissidents', Peter Duesberg and David Rasnick in early 2000. Later in the year, he convened a panel of international experts to help South Africa find 'an African solution' to the AIDS crisis. Nearly half of them didn't believe that HIV caused AIDS. Mbeki himself argues, 'You cannot attribute immune deficiency solely and exclusively to a virus.'[7] In September 2000, South African Health Minister Manto Tshabalala-Msimang circulated some of Mr Cooper's conspiracy theories to senior health officials.

The truth about AIDS is more banal. The epidemic spreads rapidly in a population when lots of heterosexual people have lots of risky sex. This is what has happened in Africa. It's a sensitive subject. People are defensive about sex and morality. Do Africans have more partners than people from other parts of the world? Researchers seem to have steered clear of the subject, fearful that their work might be labelled racist. Hein Marais, a South African journalist writes,

'Illuminating this blind spot would mean traversing the field of age-old white myths and anxieties about black sexuality, terrain few researchers are willing to venture onto.'[8]

The picture is complex. A UNAIDS report in 2000 reveals that Africans tend to start having sex younger and African girls become sexually active at a younger age than boys.[9] Elsewhere, the reverse is true. Highly biologically vulnerable in their teens, girls are getting infected in their earliest sexual experiences. In regions where there are more sexually active young people than married ones, the epidemic has been worse. The report alludes to the issue of increased risk through multiple partners and overlapping relationships, quoting a survey in rural Kenya where the average number of pre-marital partners for men was nine and for women was three.

Patterns of 'sexual networking' in Africa are also different, and more dangerous, than in other places. There is more sexual contact between people of different generations. To simplify, middle-aged men seek young partners, who they believe are less likely to be HIV-positive. Schoolgirls, tempted by the gifts lavished on them by 'sugar daddies', often succumb. Many are thus already infected by the time they marry. They pass the virus on to their husbands, who in turn infect their younger mistresses. And so the cycle continues. Contrast this with the scenario more typical of Asian countries: a husband may contract HIV from a prostitute and give it to his wife, who will then perhaps infect her unborn child. But the cycle stops there (unless he then infects other prostitutes). In Asian and Islamic countries, the taboo against premarital sex for women is more strictly enforced than it is in much of Africa, which is surely a reason why AIDS has spread more slowly in such countries.

The shortage of data on sexual behaviour, and public discussion of research that does exist, is striking, given that a sexually transmitted epidemic has been raging since the 1980s. Anecdotally, and off-the-record, doctors, epidemiologists and non-governmental organisation (NGO) workers will, without a trace of judgement, talk about how many partners their clients have. Some of the more macho truck drivers at Beitbridge, on the border between South Africa and Zimbabwe, boast about having sex with up to 30 women a month. Their partners are usually prostitutes, and they only sometimes use condoms. It is the social norm. Given the nature of their job, truckers have more opportunity for casual sex than most. But they are not the only group whose members earn a regular income and spend a long time away from home.

Africa's poverty has accelerated the spread of AIDS. Many Africans simply cannot afford to protect themselves. They can't afford condoms or antibiotics to treat other sexually transmitted diseases, which are rife in Africa. This is important because a person's risk of getting HIV dramatically increases if they have a genital discharge or ulcers. The virus enters the body more easily through open sores and inflamed mucosal surfaces.

Poor people often have little choice but to undertake dangerous jobs. Too many African women can survive only by prostituting themselves, and clients will sometimes pay double for unprotected sex. Too many African men have to travel far from home to seek work in gold mines or as truckers. Such displacement destabilises sexual relationships and helps spread the virus. Miners in southern Africa may be separated from their wives for many months a year. Many sleep with the prostitutes who congregate around miners' hostels. It is hard to persuade a poor person, or one in a dangerous job like mining, 'to give up an orgasm today so that they can, in ten years' time, prolong their enjoyment of endemic unemployment, poverty and conflict'.[10]

Africa's seemingly endless wars help spread the virus, too. Soldiers enjoy regular pay and consequently the opportunity to buy sex. The civil war in the Democratic Republic of Congo, for example, involved at least 14 separate armies and rebel factions in 2000. In the healthiest of these marauding hordes, about half of the soldiers were estimated to be HIV-positive. Among Zimbabwean troops in the Congo, the figure was perhaps 80 per cent.[11] The devastation that these armies leave in their wake, as they cut, shoot and rape their way through the Congolese jungle, can only be guessed at. Waves of refugees from this and other conflicts continue to ferry the virus *en masse* across Africa's porous borders.

Asking anyone in these situations to abstain from sex or be monogamous is unrealistic. By far the best prevention method available is condoms. However, even where they're freely available, the weight of custom makes it hard for many African women to insist that their husbands or boyfriends use them. They have little bodily autonomy, and rape is sadly too common.

No one *likes* condoms. But in Africa, it's Russian roulette to have sex without one. Despite this, many men refuse to 'condomise'. Some because they want lots of children. Others because they feel that rubber diminishes their pleasure, or because they're drunk or because they think condoms too expensive or unreliable. A batch distributed by the South African government had to be recalled because they had been stapled to leaflets. Some believe that contraception is somehow 'unAfrican' or that the white man is promoting condoms to reduce the African birth rate.

There are a number of cultural practices that have contributed to the spread of AIDS in Africa. Men in some areas were obliged to marry and provide for their recently deceased brother's widow. If the man died of AIDS, the virus is likely to be passed from his infected wife to his brother and sister-in-law. Traditional healers used unsterilised razors to perform circumcisions and to cut ritual scars on people's cheeks. But in the last decade these customs have lost popularity, as people have learned of the dangers. However, a recent reported rise in child rape in South Africa has been attributed to the myth that a man can rid himself of HIV by sleeping with a virgin.

African governments have done too little, too late. Most lack the money and the political will to improve sex education in schools or to hand out more condoms. They may try to provide health care to their citizens, but there are never enough clinics, nurses or drugs.

The epidemic didn't happen overnight, but its spread was insidiously invisible. 'For too long we have closed our eyes, hoping the truth was not so real ... ' said Thabo Mbeki, then Deputy President, in 1998. It was the first major speech about AIDS by such a senior South African politician. It was at least eight years too late.

Many Africans still do not know the facts about AIDS. Such ignorance is not exclusive to Africa, but it matters more when HIV prevalence is so high. Many Africans have missed out on safe sex messages because they didn't get enough schooling to be able to read leaflets or newspapers and they can't afford a television or radio. Many don't understand how a virus spreads or how a condom blocks it.

Even in places where most people have now heard of it, it's spoken of in euphemisms like 'this thing'. Many Africans are not changing their sexual behaviour because they don't perceive themselves to be at risk. A study in Carletonville, a mining town in South Africa, found that a fifth of those who didn't consider themselves at any risk were, in fact, infected.[12] As long as people believe that AIDS only happens to other groups – gay men, prostitutes, drug addicts, whites, blacks – they are unlikely to change their sexual behaviour.

How is AIDS affecting Africa? At household level, it's been catastrophic. AIDS kills people at their productive peak, and often more than one person in the same family. Breadwinners sicken and die.

Children, especially girls, drop out of school to take over adult roles in the home. Health care and funeral costs soar. AIDS-afflicted households sink further into poverty.

Currently, most developing countries' populations form a pyramid, with lots of children at the base, and only a few old people at the top. As AIDS thins the middle generation, this pyramid will become a 'chimney': lots of children at the bottom, a fair number of elderly at the top, and precious few middle-aged people in the middle to support them all.[13]

AIDS is unlikely to cause the total number of people in the world to shrink. Even in Africa, where AIDS is now the biggest cause of death, births still far exceed deaths. But in some badly-affected countries with relatively low fertility rates, like Zimbabwe, South Africa and Botswana, AIDS will cause populations to decline by 0.1–0.3 per cent per annum, from about 2003. Without AIDS, they would have grown by 1–3 per cent a year. This is the first time that negative population growth has been projected for developing countries.[14]

There is no doubt that AIDS will make Africans poorer. The impact of AIDS on gross domestic product will be significant, but not as awful as it is on households. As with the demographic impact, the effect of AIDS on African economies can only be guessed at. In many countries, it is unskilled workers who are most likely to die of AIDS. In economies suffering high unemployment, the vacancies so created are easily filled. However, skilled employees are also dying, and they will be harder to replace. ING Barings, an investment bank, has estimated that at the peak of South Africa's AIDS epidemic, around 2010, more than 1 per cent of highly skilled workers and 3 per cent of unskilled workers will be dying annually.[15] Even when losing this many staff, most businesses will probably be able to weather the storm. But the costs will be cumulatively vast.

The World Bank estimates that when 8 per cent of adults become infected in a country, as has already happened in 21 African countries, per capita growth rates are reduced by 0.4 per cent per annum. Given the continent's already sluggish rate of expansion, barely matching population growth in most countries, that's quite a loss.[16]

So what's being done to curb the epidemic? Very little, by most developing countries' governments. Uganda, Senegal and Thailand are notable exceptions.

In Uganda, where the rate has dropped from about 14 per cent in the early 1990s to about 8 per cent now, President Yoweri Museveni has talked frankly about AIDS since the late 1980s and created an environment where NGOs feel free to offer explicit sex education without asking anyone's permission and without encountering official resistance.[17]

In 1993, Catharine Watson started *Straight Talk*, a magazine aimed at 16–18 year old Ugandans that deals with everything from relationships to masturbation. They don't just tell readers, 'Use condoms': they explain how the virus lives in sexual fluids, and how a condom can catch these fluids.

> 'Later, we launched *Young Talk* for 10–14 year olds,' says Catharine, 'and posted it to every primary school. After a couple of months, we sent a package of back issues to the Minister of Education, who's now the Prime Minister, explaining what we do. He wrote back saying he was proud to be involved ... The government can't do everything.'

She's had visitors from NGOs in Zimbabwe who can't believe that *Straight Talk* staff are allowed to do what they're doing.

In Thailand, the government launched a '100 per cent condom use' campaign for commercial sex, which dramatically slowed the spread of the disease. The Senegalese government undertook a similar campaign, and managed to contain the epidemic before it got a hold. Condom use there soared from 800,000 in 1988 to seven million in 1997 and HIV prevalence has stayed below 2 per cent.

What works? Making noise. A president's every word is broadcast on national television, so if he slips a 'safe sex' message into every speech, it will eventually sink in.

Governments have also helped by simply letting NGOs get on with their job. Where they have placed prudish restrictions on NGOs, the message is stifled. Kenyan President Daniel arap Moi, for instance, did not allow condoms to be promoted until 1999, for fear of upsetting traditionalist Catholics.

Governments must strive to provide the best public health service possible, given limited resources. The anti-retroviral drug cocktails used in the West are impossibly expensive for most Africans. Even with discounts, they cost thousands of dollars each year, putting them out of reach of all but tycoons and cabinet ministers. But there are several cheaper treatments that can save lives. Basic medicines for opportunistic infections such as tuberculosis and malaria can make a big difference. Treating other sexually transmitted diseases slows the spread of the virus, usually with simple antibiotics. Voluntary HIV testing and counselling are useful.

For the richer African countries, a relatively cheap anti-retroviral drug called Nevirapine can actually save money as well as lives. A single dose given to an HIV-positive pregnant woman reduces the chance that she will pass the virus to her baby. A child with AIDS costs much more to care for. More controversially, African countries could consider legalising abortion. Currently, only South Africa allows it.

Finally, making friends with foreign donors helps. Most African governments depend on foreign money to pay for AIDS control programmes. Governments can encourage donations by being open about how they are spent, or they can alienate donors by treating every query as a violation of national sovereignty.

What hasn't worked? Endless talkshops. Governments frequently form new committees to discuss AIDS. 'Stakeholders' are consulted. 'Multi-sectoral' strategies are drafted. Only when plans are put into practice can they make a difference.

Some governments have also wasted precious time reinventing the wheel. In South Africa, for instance, President Thabo Mbeki has questioned the scientific consensus around AIDS. In 1997, he backed Virodene, a local 'cure' that was in fact an industrial solvent, and purged the South African drug regulatory agency when it objected. In 1999, he declared that AZT (a drug that has been licensed around the world for over a decade) is too dangerous to prescribe for HIV-positive pregnant women. And in 2000, he questioned the link between HIV and AIDS. The result? Confusion. Some South Africans now believe they don't need to use condoms because they think Mr Mbeki is saying that AIDS doesn't exist.

Prevention campaigns can work. In 1990, South Africa and Thailand both had HIV prevalence rates amongst pregnant women of less than 1 per cent. By 1998, South Africa's epidemic was out of control at 23 per cent, but Thailand's had only risen to 1.5 per cent.

Organisations doing preventive work normally target high-risk groups such as sex workers, miners, truckers and young people. They offer condoms, videos, leaflets and antibiotics for sexually transmitted diseases. They often use 'peer educators' (prostitutes to teach other prostitutes) on the assumption that they will be trusted more than outsiders would be. Young people are taught 'life skills', such as how to insist that their partners use condoms. Condoms (including the new female condom) are marketed like commercial products, with energetic advertising and fancy packaging. They are usually subsidised, but not free, because people are more likely to use and trust what they pay for.

Anything that alleviates poverty helps, too. If governments help poor people to build homes for themselves, or start up small businesses, this might encourage them to take fewer sexual risks, because they have more to lose.

With hospitals overflowing, organisations are arranging 'home-based care' as the only hope of supporting the vast numbers of AIDS-affected families. Volunteers visit homes to offer counselling and pass on basic nursing tips to family members. Some NGOs are trying to teach orphans how to avoid contracting the disease themselves, at the same time as they teach them how to look after their sick parents. If they can't get hold of rubber gloves, they're shown how to tie plastic bags onto their small hands with elastic bands.

Why is there an AIDS orphan crisis in Africa? Apart from the obvious answer that AIDS has killed large numbers of adults of parenting age, most Africans like to have big families. It offers status and acts as an insurance policy; your children will look after you in old age. Consequently, when African parents die, they leave lots of orphans. Ugandan women, for instance, had an average of seven children in 1998, and Zambian women had an average of five or six. Compare this with Thai, Chinese, British and Italian women who had an average of between one and two children.[18]

Many African parents are no longer living long enough to see their children reach maturity. Weakened by malnutrition, HIV-positive Africans tend to sicken and die faster than HIV-positive Westerners. They can't afford enough food, clean drinking water and the drugs to treat opportunistic infections, let alone the cocktails of anti-retroviral drugs that keep HIV-positive North Americans and Europeans alive for years. Activists are fighting to get drug companies to offer discounts to poor countries. But even if they succeed, few African clinics are equipped to administer such treatments. Drug-resistant strains of the virus and a black market in drugs siphoned out of public health systems would swiftly emerge if patients' adherence to complex drug regimens and the distribution of drug supplies are not carefully monitored.

The African extended family has traditionally nursed its sick, and absorbed its orphans without fuss or legal process. In most cases, it still does. In some African countries, it remains the only safety net for orphans. The state often has no money to offer alternatives like orphanages, grants for foster parents or salaries and bicycles for community volunteers.

Sometimes sibling groups are split up between aunts and uncles in order to share the cost, but somehow or other, the African extended family continues to shoulder the burden. In all heavily affected countries, there is now an army of grandmothers, aunts and older sisters struggling to care for exploding numbers of orphans. But as the pressure on them grows, they are going to need help in order to feed those extra mouths.

Inevitably, some families are collapsing. In the most desperate cases, relatives steal orphans' inheritances. Some children struggle on alone in their parents' house. These child-headed households are a new phenomenon. If they're lucky a neighbour may check that they're eating. If nobody cares, they may end up on the streets.

What's being done for the orphans? Every government, except Somalia and the US, has ratified the Convention on the Rights of the Child, which was adopted by the United Nations in 1989. Signatories have, at least on paper, accepted their responsibility towards their country's children. As well as the right to a basic standard of living, education, health, social security and time to play, they have also promised children protection against abuse or neglect. If a child is deprived of a family, the state must ensure that there is alternative care such as 'foster placement, kafalah of Islamic law, adoption or if necessary placement in suitable institutions' (Article 20).

But making rights a reality is much harder. Signatories are only committed to working 'in accordance with national conditions and within their means' and many other worthy causes compete for attention and scant resources. AIDS orphans are not particularly organised or vocal lobbyists.

The knee-jerk reaction to an orphan crisis might be to build orphanages. Thankfully, governments have not rushed to do this. Children rarely thrive in such places. Even when staff are loving, and donations from overseas churches ensure that their charges are well fed, institutional life can be grim. In any case, the number of AIDS orphans is going to be so large that the cost of building and maintaining orphanages would be prohibitive.

But what are the alternatives? People agree that the best place for children is in a family. If this is not possible, the next best thing is to provide some form of care within their community of origin, making sure that siblings are kept together. If this is not possible, a loving family outside their community or, as a last resort, residential care. Child abuse can occur in any setting.

Governments can help by educating people about AIDS, to try to erase the stigma. Fewer HIV-positive mothers would then abandon their babies and fewer relatives would ostracise their orphaned nieces and nephews. Governments can encourage families to foster unrelated children by publicising the fact that there are orphans needing homes, and if budgets allow, providing financial assistance, through cash benefits, food parcels or credit to start small businesses. If they can't afford to train and employ social workers to run such programmes, they should subsidise (or, at the very least, applaud) the work of NGOs, and help smooth the path for money to flow from foreign donors to grassroots organisations working with orphans and their guardians.

This book focuses on the impact of AIDS on families and speculates on the long-term effect on African society. Africa's AIDS orphans could grow up to become vulnerable and volatile adults. Some will learn to survive through theft or prostitution, numbing their pain perhaps by sniffing glue.

African countries face a stark choice. If they do not find ways to care for the growing multitude of AIDS orphans, they could soon find their streets crowded with angry, intoxicated adolescents. Besides being a human tragedy, this could aggravate the continent's already high levels of crime.

In South Africa, for instance, crime is so rampant that the rich live behind razor wire and the poor often form vigilante groups. As waves of orphans with no family and no livelihood hit the streets, it could get worse. The average age of the population is also getting younger.[19] By 2010, a quarter of South Africans will be between 14 and 24 years old, the peak ages for offending. This fact, combined with more orphans growing up in poverty and without care and guidance, will surely result in there being more young people tempted into criminal activity. Left on their own to survive, or to be exploited and abused, these children may feel that they owe society nothing.

Little is known about what happens to grown-up street children. They are hard to track into adulthood because they are such a mobile group. Some will not survive to maturity. In 1998, a fifth of the boys over ten, using the Othandweni mobile clinic for street children in Hillbrow, the decaying centre of Johannesburg, were HIV-positive.[20] If HIV prevention messages are not incorporated into projects aimed at reaching street children, and other out-of-school AIDS orphans, the epidemic will probably not be curbed within a generation.

Many people working in the AIDS field dislike the phrase 'AIDS orphan'. They worry that it stigmatises children. Much time is spent debating alternatives such as 'vulnerable and needy children', 'children in distress', 'children infected or affected by HIV/AIDS', 'children who are in need of special care and protection' and so on. For the sake of simplicity, this book will use 'AIDS orphan'. It is AIDS that is causing the crisis.

Across Africa there are many compassionate individuals who, recognising the scale of the crisis, are striving to make a difference. But currently too little is being done. The magnitude of Africa's AIDS orphan crisis calls for urgent attention from African governments, NGOs and international donors. With better planning and more aid, a high proportion of orphans can be saved from lives of misery and deprivation. If the problem is ignored, however, the consequences both for the orphans and for society will be ghastly.

Like the virus itself, the AIDS crisis mutates rapidly. New research is published, new drugs are tested and more governments wake up to the urgency of the problem. This book provides a snapshot of the circumstances of AIDS orphans in sub-Saharan Africa at the turn of the millennium. It will give an insight into those whose lives have already been scarred by the epidemic and will put some faces to the horrifying statistics.

Section I

Families

1
Mbuya's Story

A Grandmother's Story, Lusaka, Zambia

Five of old Mary Banda's eight children have died. How does she explain her family's misfortune? 'My children didn't die from any disease like this AIDS. Jealous villagers bewitched them.'

It was a long parade to the graveyard. Once a year, for five years running, she buried another of her children. The lines on her face deepened with each one. She'd always thought that, by raising eight children, she'd insured herself against hardship in old age. She was wrong. By 2000, she had inherited the task of rearing eight of her children's children. Mrs Banda has become one of Zambia's 'elderly orphaned'. The offspring she expected to look after her in her twilight years are gone. She has a throng of new dependants and no income.

Named after the Zambezi River when it gained independence in 1964, Zambia is landlocked between eight other nations in south central Africa. Zambia is peaceful, but poor. Only a few British colonists ever settled there, and unlike in neighbouring Zimbabwe or Congo, the transition to independence was relatively tranquil. Since independence, Zambia has avoided the kind of civil wars that plague the region. Its first president, Kenneth Kaunda, set up a one-party state, but it was a fairly easy-going one. Mr Kaunda was neither bloodthirsty nor personally corrupt. But his economic policies were ruinous. He nationalised everything from the great copper mines in the north to the bicycle repair shops in Lusaka. By the early 1990s, Zambia was poorer than it had been at independence. International pressure forced Mr Kaunda to hold multiparty elections, which he lost. The victor, a former union leader named Frederick Chiluba, was expected to revive Zambia's fortunes. Sadly, he has not been successful. The new regime is generally considered more competent than the previous one, but also more corrupt.

Zambia is arid and sparsely populated. Most of its ten million people are extremely poor. Perhaps three-quarters of them survive on less than $1 a day and nearly half the children are stunted from malnutrition. The state provides no safety net. The government has little money, so can't dish out pensions or child support grants to those too poor to feed and clothe themselves.

AIDS in Zambia is widespread. According to the US Bureau of the Census, it had reduced life expectancy to 37 by 1998. It would have been 56 in a world without AIDS. No one knows how many children have been orphaned. The United States Agency for International Development (USAID) estimated that in 1990, 9 per cent of children under 15 had lost their mother or both parents, maybe 61 per cent of them bereaved by AIDS. By 2000, 12 per cent had lost their mother or both parents, 76 per cent to AIDS. If paternal deaths are added into the equation, nearly a third of Zambia's children may have been affected.

Most of the children who have lost both parents are taken in by their extended family, usually by someone who is elderly, female and widowed. Research by the United Nations Children's Fund (UNICEF) revealed that nearly 40 per cent of them are cared for by grandparents (usually grandmothers) and another 30 per cent are looked after by uncles or aunts (usually their mother's sister). In towns, where half of Zambians live, orphans are more likely to be taken in by aunts or uncles. If the child lives in the countryside, she's more likely to be in a grandmother's custody. In countries like Zambia, where a fifth of the adult population are HIV-positive, grandmothers often find themselves grieving for more than one child and looking after several orphans.

Mrs Banda can't remember which year she was born, but she looks about 65. She's shy and greets visitors with a bob and timid handshake. She speaks Nyanja, the most common language in Zambia, and lives in Chuunga, a township in the Northwest outskirts of Lusaka, Zambia's capital.

'I came to the city, from a village near Malawi, when I'd just got married. My husband was a security guard. He worked for a long time with one company and made enough money to build this house. Then he died.'

Her roots in the rural area where she grew up have withered. Like many of her generation that moved to the cities, she now feels at home in Lusaka and has little contact with far-flung relatives. She's grown suspicious of villagers because she believes them to be jealous of town folk like her family.

Her home is a small, brick house with a corrugated roof. At the back, there's a small patch of well-tended vegetables. Inside, it's dark except for a shard of sunlight through a small, high window. Strips of fabric separate three rooms. At night, three grandsons sleep head to toe in a small double bed in one room. Three others sleep in a bed in the kitchen and Mrs Banda and the two girls sleep on the ground in the front room.

The orphans range in age from six to 20. Five of them – Mapala, 19, Abraham, 15, James, ten, Ruth, twelve and Eva aged six – sit silently around their grandmother's knees on the bare floor as she lists their losses.

'My only son, the oldest of my eight children, Tamanga died first. He didn't have any children. Then there was Jennifer, and she also died. Her children are Mapala and Chikabvemka. My third child was Olio, mother of Abraham and David. My fourth child was Anna. She died leaving two children but they're staying with other relatives. Malawi, my fifth child, had Ruth, Eva, James and Bernard.

'I nursed my children until the illness got really bad and I couldn't cope any more. Then I took them to the hospital where they died. They were dying – one, two, three, four, five – in the order they were born. But, you know, I can't remember how old they were when they died. I keep forgetting things.'

Mrs Banda is adamant that they were all struck down by witchcraft. The grandchildren roll their eyes when she's talking about it, but not so she can see. They clearly don't believe in the witchcraft theory, but they wouldn't dream of contradicting her.

Belief in witchcraft is widespread in Africa. In a study of AIDS orphans in Kenya in 1999, nearly a third of them believed that their parents had died because of witchcraft or *chira* (a curse).

'They died because they were successful', explains Mrs Banda. 'My four daughters were businesswomen. They used to buy second-hand clothes here in Lusaka and exchange them for groundnuts in the village, which they'd sell back in town. Jealous villagers bewitched them through their feet. First they got pains in their legs, and then in their chests and later, they had headaches. That's how my girls died. And Tamanga was promoted at work and given a car, so jealous people put medicine on the brake or something in the engine, so it got in through his feet and he got sick and died.'

AIDS is an unpredictable disease. Sometimes you feel healthy, but sooner or later you suffer a series of frightening symptoms. Sometimes you cannot breathe. Sometimes you cough up blood. In quick succession you may suffer skin and mouth infections, fever, rigid muscles, convulsions, depression and delirium. This can last for two years or more. During the disease's terminal stage, which may last for up to a year, you may be bedridden, incontinent, wasted and suffer dementia. Your appearance and personality may change.

When breadwinners sicken, families can rapidly become impoverished as they use up their savings and sell off their possessions to pay for health care and funerals.

'When my children became sick,' says Mrs Banda, 'I took them to traditional healers, as well as to the hospital. It was the witchdoctors who told me they'd been bewitched in the village, but they didn't say by whom. The government has made a ruling that traditional healers shouldn't tell people that so-and-so bewitched their child because it causes fights.'

Mrs Banda is remarkably matter-of-fact about all this. She's not angry. She doesn't want justice, compensation or revenge. She's resigned.

'*Mbuyas* [grandmothers] like me must try not to be bitter that people have killed our children and now we have to look after orphans. We shouldn't try and seek vengeance on those people. Vengeance is for the Lord.'

Mrs Banda believes there are ways to protect yourself against jealousy. If only her children had followed her advice.

'The first thing to do is go and visit a witchdoctor. They advertise on radio. They'll give you medicine you can put on your feet so that even if you're bewitched in the villages, it's not going to work. Anyone wanting to do business should avoid doing it in their home village because they're bound to be jealous there ... '

Ten-year-old James sniggers when his granny loses her train of thought and says, 'I've forgotten what I was talking about. I keep forgetting things now.'

'I used to just look after two grandchildren,' she continues, 'because it's traditional in Zambia to keep some grandchildren even when their parents are alive. But when my children started dying, all these other children started moving in. It was OK at first because my other offspring were helping. The real problems began when I no longer had children able to help, and more and more grandchildren needing to move in.'

The children barely speak. They look depressed. At times, one will rest his head on his arms. It's impossible to know what they're thinking as their granny talks about how hard her life has become. Only James smiles. The older ones just look weary.

It seems to be a relief for Mrs Banda to talk about her woes.

'My three surviving daughters can't help much,' she says without obvious resentment. 'My youngest, Mabvuto is here in Lusaka but she's unemployed. Esimaga married a South African guerrilla who was here during the struggle for an independent South Africa about six years ago and we haven't seen her since. I think she's in South Africa. Sarah's married but she doesn't work and her husband only gets pieces of work here and there. She tries to help us by coming round with a bag of mealie meal [maize] or beans.

'The children's biggest problem is getting enough food. Sometimes I sell groundnuts by the road. Those who are feeling sorry give me some money. But it's not enough. We try to grow some maize, sweet potato and greens so we have two meals a day. The older boys have been very helpful in the garden. They don't mind. When my children were sick I couldn't go to the fields, so they were doing most of the work then. And Ruth helps me with the cooking and washing plates and taking care of little Eva.

'Only James and Ruth are in school and even they are sometimes chased away because they don't have shoes, fees or uniforms.'

Mrs Banda looks in good health, but her smallest grandchild, Eva is sick. She's feverish and has been hallucinating. Her eyes are glazed and she lies across her sister's legs, whimpering. Eventually she leaves the group to go and lie down next door. She can be heard coughing.

'All I can do is just keep cutting firewood and putting it into the brazier to keep the home warm', says Mrs Banda anxiously. 'I can't even afford to buy blankets to cover her when she's shivering, let alone medicines.'

Three grandsons – Chikabvemka, 20, David, 19 and Bernard, 18 – are also ill at the moment but an uncle has taken them to a local clinic.

Mrs Banda isn't entirely on her own.

'I like to go to church and meet my friends. We share problems, and it makes you realise you're not the only one. There are lots of people in the same position as me.

'I also get help from an organisation called Children in Distress Widows' Support Group. Once a month they give me some mealie meal [maize], beans and cooking oil, but it's not enough because the boys are eating all the time. When all the deaths were happening, friends from church would cook for the people coming to the funerals. Neighbours raised some money to get a few planks to make up the coffins, and some women from Children in Distress came and comforted me.'

Mrs Banda's grandchildren are in some ways quite fortunate. They have love, companionship and a crowded, but safe, place to sleep. But they rarely have enough to eat and they go barefoot to school, or not at all. And they have no parents. Sickness, death and poverty have scarred their youth.

'I'm an old woman who's suffering', says Mrs Banda. 'When I was young, I never thought such cruel things could happen. When I think about it, I pray and cry, but I don't like to cry because it'll upset the children. The church has given me the strength to go on because I know that one day I'll die too and join my children.'

In Zambia, the surviving family of someone who's died of AIDS will not be shunned as they might be in some other countries. The disease is so common that it has lost much of its social stigma. But people still do not like to talk about it publicly. John Munsanje, who runs the head office of Children in Distress, a non-governmental organisation (NGO) that helps widows, grandmothers and orphans, observes,

'You can tell that grandmothers are not keen to say the word "AIDS", but they know what it is. There's still a hangover of a feeling that it's an immoral disease because it's transmitted sexually. They may use another language or euphemism like "*kaliyondeyonde*" (slim) or "*Aya maitenda yatu*" (This very disease). Grandmothers, especially, may say, "It's like the *kauka* (worm) was eating up someone", or "The *chinyoni* (big bird) is about to grab that person." It's a way of avoiding it. They're not open, but it's getting easier.'

Social workers duck the issue, too. They don't know what the grandmothers they look after were told at the hospital. They can't assume that clients know that their children died of AIDS and they don't want to add to the trauma. Mrs Banda, for instance, has no idea that she gets food parcels because they've identified her as needy because AIDS has killed so many of her family. She claims she's never met anyone with the disease.

NGOs like Children in Distress target assistance to widows. Far fewer widowers need food parcels or emotional support because they tend to remarry quickly and can generally rely on the support of their mothers and sisters. Widows, however, find it almost impossible to find another husband.

Children in Distress has branches called 'widows' support groups' throughout Zambia. Each was started when a few women in an area got together and compared notes. John explains,

'It'll usually be a religiously motivated person or an individual overwhelmed with the orphan situation in her own family who comes to you. I say to her, "You are one. There are others. How do you think you can deal with this problem?" They then begin to recognise that collectively they can cope better. Once a spark of initiative has been shown, we pitch in with encouragement and offer them training courses. Naturally their expectations grow from when we come in, so we need to be very candid about what we can provide. I tell them that they have to recognise the resources that are around them, human resources if not material. When a group takes off, its members find themselves with a shoulder to cry on and a monthly food parcel for those who really need it.

'When a family's struggling, the wider community should pitch in and help,' says John. 'The best way for outsiders to help is through organisations based in the community. That's what our widows' groups are.'

The parent NGO in this sort of arrangement often has to take care that no local branch grows too dependent on it. If they are to survive, each group has to raise its own money and maintain its own momentum. It is also important to make sure that no individual member becomes wholly dependent on food parcels. Poor people are usually delighted to receive handouts, but handouts can never be a long-term solution. Children in Distress are beginning to train members in business skills. Staff are being taught how to manage credit schemes to kick start their members' small businesses.

John has no illusions about how difficult it will be introducing the idea of loans that need to be repaid, when most of their clients don't have enough to eat.

'We have to start somewhere so members realise that eventually they're going to have to face reality and find their own food. At the moment you can tell that, because of destitution, they really have to get food and they're not aware of the danger of handouts. It's going to take a long time but they need to manage their own lives in the end.'

Meanwhile, desperate *mbuyas* are queuing up to join Children in Distress.

'The food programme has to be run locally', explains John. 'Branches appoint a social welfare committee who go round and identify the really needy. They look at the living conditions, if there are grandparents, how many children, how young are the children, how many are sick and whether it's a child-headed household. But of course there are a few incidents where a committee member's relative benefits instead of the most needy. Our members are human, I'm afraid.

'Amongst our members, we don't have a single grandmother who's found the energy to really start life again and get a business off the ground. If I saw one I'd use her as a role model. It's difficult for them. They expected to be looked after so they're pitying themselves and mourning their lost sons and daughters. You see tears drop when they're reminded of what's happened to them. The only thing that pleases them is seeing the children. But even then, there's not much hope because they know their future's insecure because they're not in school now.'

For orphans, the good thing about living with their grandmother is that she loves them and treats them all equally. The downside is that their material deprivation, and their grandmother's, often worsens. Expecting a grandmother to become a dynamic business-woman in her seventies is unrealistic. She's sad and tired.

John ponders the relative merits of grandmothers and aunts.

'Grannies are the fairest guardians. An aunt is more likely to dis-criminate slightly in favour of her own children. And her husband may resent the extra mouths to feed.

'But if I had to choose, I think it's better for an orphan to go to an auntie because she's usually got more money. Also, grannies are bad at disciplining children. You never get fierce grandmoth-ers. They want to be nice.'

Mrs Banda worries about her grandchildren getting into trouble, but she believes that she has found a method to keep an eye on them by insisting that they come home for one meal a day.

'It's difficult dealing with grown-up children', she admits. 'There are temptations. They like to roam about. But what I try to do to keep them in order is to always make sure, even if there is very little food, that I cook for them and that we sit down and eat it together. Otherwise they'd be running around and falling into mischief. Especially the boys.

'I worry that Ruth could be tempted, you know, to play around with boys. She's twelve. She's growing up and she thinks she's a beautiful girl. I'm strict. I've told her not to play in the night. If there's a man who wants to marry her, that man should come and present himself in broad daylight.'

Methods of discipline have changed in the family. Mrs Banda treats Eva, the youngest, differently.

'Usually Zambian people would whip their kids of Eva's age if they do something naughty, but I don't in her case, because she would think, "Oh God, somebody's whipping me because I don't have parents." So even if she does something wrong, I talk and play with her instead of hitting her.

'I like to tell the children stories and share my thoughts with them. I tell them that they must respect people with grey hair, like myself. And when they see an elderly man, they must respect him and see him like a father. And any elderly woman is like a mother. I also tell them they must respect other people's property. Otherwise, if they are playing around and stealing, they are going to be killed and they won't even grow up.'

She gives them sage advice but can't enforce her rules because she hasn't got the energy.

'Most *mbuyas* were kept by the children who died so they remain dependent and frail', says John Munsanje. 'They don't expect much from the children because they know they're about to go. They just worry about the children's own future. It's a tormenting thought, "What happens when I die?"'

Zambia's Public Welfare Assistance System is meant to provide a safety net for the destitute amongst the unemployed, old, orphaned and disabled. It doesn't. John is on the district committee that decides who in the capital is poor enough to be helped. He explains how it operates,

'Applicants go to the district office and say, "I'm an orphan and I'm struggling to feed myself." The officers register the case, do a home visit and go to the school. It takes time because they have so many applicants and just a few, very demotivated staff. How far can they get when they don't have a car and cover a huge area? How can they determine whether people are telling the truth? It's guesswork.'

Once the haphazard screening's completed, the reports go before the committee that decides who gets what. Applicants are rarely rejected. The system rewards those who know their way around it, were quick to ask for help, able to fill out a form and lucky enough to get their application processed. If you're related to a civil servant, your chance of getting help from the state increases dramatically.

The district office may pay an orphan's school fees or a social worker may go with the client to buy medicine for them. Food is occasionally given out to the elderly. Cash, never. John says,

'We've persuaded a lot of grandmothers to be repatriated to rural areas, because we believe it's easier for them to survive there.

Although drought is a problem. We say, "Please go home." They're allowed to settle anywhere. They don't have to go to their original village. We even provide transport money for them, and maybe a bit of assistance to get them started. For instance, one of them might say, "Buy me a bag of salt, which I can use to exchange for labour to get a plot of land ploughed."

'Of course, the system can't cover everyone. There's so little money. We have to say, "We'll give this. Too bad for the rest." It's hard.'

Few people even know that a bag of salt and some painkillers may be available from the state. It's not well advertised. If it were, there would be trouble. They are already overwhelmed with applicants. Basically, Zambia's poor are on their own, unless they belong to supportive community groups or churches.

Even without the epidemic, many elderly Zambians would struggle. Rapid urbanisation has weakened family ties. Young adults often live far from the villages where their parents remain. City life is more individualistic than village life. Many modern urbanites feel less duty-bound to support their parents than rural traditions would require. Rising divorce rates splinter families still further.

AIDS is accelerating the breakdown of the traditional African family. Grandmothers have always been involved in the socialisation of their grandchildren, enabling many mothers to leave their children for long periods in order to find work and support all three generations. AIDS orphans are going to raise their own children without the loving support and free childcare that grandmothers used to provide. Perhaps they will choose to have fewer children. The children of AIDS orphans will never know the love of grandparents. And the *mbuyas* now? As Zambia's middle generation dies, grandmothers are left holding the baby.

2
Extended Families

An Aunt's Story, Kampala, Uganda

When Susan Nagawa died of AIDS someone had to look after her children. Her sister, Sophia Mukasa-Monico, already had two of her own, but she knew her duty. She returned to Uganda, from Italy where she'd been living for over a decade, to adopt her orphaned teenage niece and nephew, Sharrot and Sandy. That was in 1990. Since then her home in the capital, Kampala, has filled up. With Sharrot and Sandy came another six teenagers, the orphans of Susan's co-wives. When AIDS strikes a polygamous family, things can get complicated.

Uganda is a lush, green country in East Africa, but its people are poor. In Kampala, Marabou storks, the size of children, fly overhead. They arrived during President Idi Amin's rule (1971–79), when as many as 350,000 people were murdered by the state. Corpses rotted in the streets. Even more Ugandans were killed under President Milton Obote (1962–71 and 1980–85). Since 1986, things have changed for the better. Now the birds just eat rubbish.

Although Uganda is now more peaceful and less poor, AIDS is killing Ugandans at an alarming rate. People talk about the disease openly because every extended family has now lost someone to it. By 2000, there were nearly two million AIDS orphans. Ugandans are optimistic that their epidemic has peaked because, at last, the number of HIV-positive people appears to be decreasing, in some places by as much as half.

Sophia Mukasa-Monico is a beautiful, confident woman in her forties. She's comfortably off and lives in a two-bedroom house in the city. Her brother-in-law, and Sandy and Sharrots' father, Reginah Nagawa, was a 'Big Man'. He owned a factory that processed maize, had eleven wives (some more formally wed than others) and 22 children. But AIDS ravaged his family. Mr Nagawa died of it in 1992. Five of his wives and three of his children have died; two of the latter in infancy, one at the age of 26. The surviving 19 orphans range in age from ten to 29.

'I decided to adopt my sister's two children,' says Sophia. 'But I didn't want to completely pull them out of their big family. They used to live together in a vast house in a village in Mbarara in southwest Uganda, so they're very close. One of their father's dying wishes was that they shouldn't be separated.'

Having ten children, and children from different families, is common in Uganda. But it's hard work.

'You really do give and give', says Sophia. 'My two kids are the youngest and, at times, I feel they're missing out. It makes them demand my attention more. When there were just them and Sandy and Sharrot, we would go out and have pizza but now with six more, I can't afford it.

'I've told them, "I'm doing this but I can't pretend to substitute for your mothers, because I'm not." And I tell them that if they feel I am treating my children in a special way it's because they *are* my children. Sometimes I feel guilty ... but I talk straight to them and I think they appreciate it.

'Last holiday, Sylivia, who's 18, came to me and said, "One of our aunties said that we're weighing you down. Is it true?" And she looked me in the eye, "Is it true?" And I said, "You know, Sylivia, it's not easy but if it becomes a burden and I can't bear it, I'll tell you."'

Because the six additional children who have joined Sophia's household share no blood with her, her decision to take them on was greeted with incomprehension by many. People understand that Sophia's obliged to take in her sister's children, but the others aren't even her tribe. Friends and acquaintances ask her, 'Why do you do it? What are you going to gain from it?' But the kids appreciate what she's done, and show it by offering to cook and clean.

Sophia's Italian husband died when he was 35. She was four months pregnant with Bosco when she discovered he had cancer and he died eight months later. A lawyer by training, Sophia now runs The AIDS Support Organisation (TASO), a non-governmental organisation (NGO) that has been helping Ugandan people with AIDS and their families since 1987.

'I got involved with TASO because my husband received an amazing level of care in Italy, mostly provided by volunteers. He would call them at all times of night and they would turn up, knowing there was really nothing they could do, but they would come and just the fact that they were helping felt good.

'I joined TASO thinking I'd be a volunteer like those who used to help my husband. But they were looking for a Director!

'And my sister ... I was feeling bad that I wasn't here when Susan was dying. She wrote to me when her third kid died, and I had just gone through the death of my husband, so I told her, "Don't worry." And later she wrote and told me that her husband had AIDS, but, stupidly, I didn't imagine that she might also have it, so I told her, "Don't worry, even if he dies, we'll support each other ... " It was only after her death that I realised I could have done more for her. I hadn't known what AIDS was about. In Italy, only drug users had AIDS and you didn't really hear about it.

'So I said to myself, "To pay back this woman, I'll go back to Uganda and look after her children." And then I heard about TASO and said, "Why not? I can join this group and do something useful."'

Sophia knew nothing of the stigma that surrounded AIDS. People assumed that anyone working for TASO was HIV-positive.

'When I joined TASO, I didn't know that people were going to gossip about me. People would look at me and then look away. That's when I realised how bad things were here.

'It's no longer like that. If stigma still exists in Uganda, it's self-inflicted. A person with HIV may worry about how people are looking at them, even if they're not being looked at. And you can only get over this by talking; talking until you get to a point where you realise, "I can talk about it without anybody giving me pitying eyes." I think my niece, Sharrot, still suffers a mixture of anger and fear of pity.'

Sharrot is 14 and was adopted by Sophia when she was eight. She barely knew her mother because she was six when her mother died and during most of her early years, her mother was sick. She doesn't talk about her.

'Once when we went to see her in school she came to me saying, "Mummy, you know that teacher who's a relative of ours, she went and told the whole staff room that you aren't my mother."

And then she burst into tears. She said, "What makes me angry is that they're now looking at me with pitying eyes and I don't like it. And they all say I'm not open."'

Sophia confronted the teacher, saying, 'In the kind of world we're living in now, it's unfair to do that to a child. Sharrot knows that her mother died of AIDS, but this is how she copes. When she grows up she'll want to find out more about her mother, but this girl didn't really know her mother, and anyone who can act as a mother is most welcome. These children need a lot of help, not pity.'

Some Ugandan children have absorbed HIV prevention messages that say you can avoid AIDS by using a condom, sticking to one partner or by abstaining from sex. So they're angry with grown-ups that get AIDS and then leave them orphaned. 'At TASO, we have a book for collecting children's thoughts and the biggest feeling that comes out is anger', observes Sophia. 'They sometimes write that they hate TASO because they say TASO looks after people with AIDS, and they get better, look nice again and then go out and infect others.'

Having watched their parents waste away, one might imagine that AIDS orphans would be fastidious about safe sex. Sadly, many are not. NGO workers observe that being orphaned by AIDS actually makes children more vulnerable to becoming infected themselves.

A few of Sophia's brood are at high risk. Sixteen-year-old twins, Sheba and Sissy, have become commercial sex workers. 'They dropped out of school,' says Sophia, 'and there was no one to run after them. Their relatives and I don't have the time, so we've rented an apartment for them. During the day they come to my home to talk with their brothers. We all eat together and then they go back to their flat.'

Both girls have had abortions in the last month.

'What this shows,' says Sophia, 'is they're having unprotected sex with all kinds of men. So I told them that after what they'd gone through, I'd take them for family planning and it would be the contraceptive injection which lasts for three months a time. I'll make sure they have condoms, but I don't know if they'd be able to persuade men to use them. And then I'll take them for an HIV test.'

The twins are not the only ones in trouble. Their older brother, Ssalongo, who is 21, is in prison because he assaulted a man.

Sophia seems ambivalent about the twins. She's sympathetic, but she's not rushing in to try to rescue them. She believes in personal responsibility.

'The twins are very vulnerable but it's their choice', she says. 'Their mother died in 1989, and, since then, they've had everything the others have had. All the others have gone through the same story in their lives but they're more resilient maybe. Coping depends on the individual. But it's not easy to look after the twins and I really don't want them to mix with the others who are doing well in school.'

Fortunately, the children have a wealthy uncle who's prepared to pay for their boarding school fees. They only stay with Sophia in the school holidays. But during term time, she's still involved helping sort out their crises.

Sadic, who's 16, has been suspended from school. Sophia heard his side of the story and then went to see the headmaster who

'described a boy so different to the Sadic I know. He pointed out that maybe Sadic has problems. He joined a stupid group that think they're top of the school. Maybe he found some sort of security with them because he only moved into my home in '99 and that's when he discovered rules. Before that, he and his siblings used to come and go.

'So Sadic and I talked matters straight. People wanted me to beat him but I said, "I don't beat children." Instead I gave him the worst punishment I could think of. I stopped him going dancing with his friends. He cried like a baby. And I said, "I know it hurts, but you have to show you're a different person in school."'

One of the orphans, Sylvia, who shares a mother with the twins and Ssalongo, is doing well at school. She feels responsible for the others and sends Sophia thank-you cards on behalf of all of them. She cried when she heard that Sadic had been sent home from school in disgrace, even though he's only her half-brother.

During discussions at TASO, families who have taken in orphans frequently complain about the children's ingratitude. Some orphans mistreat their adoptive siblings or make up nasty stories about their foster parents. Sophia's never had any problems like this. She has, however, had problems with the man in her life not accepting her decision to take on the children.

'After my husband died, I had another Italian partner and a second child, Betty', she says. 'I returned to Uganda to take on my sister's children and my partner followed me. I was living with my mum initially, and he moved in with us. He hadn't lived in Uganda before and it was really hard for him.

'He moved out, but stayed in Kampala. He got a well-paid engineering job and then expected me to move in with him. I said, "Let's give it a break for one year. Try to find your own life in Uganda. And if, after that time, we still need each other, we'll get back together."

'After one year, he came back and said, "Let's try again." So I moved in with him with my two kids and my sister's two. But he didn't like it. So I said, "Let's be together, but let me go back to my mother's." For the next two years we lived apart but he'd regularly come and take out Bosco and Betty.

'Then in 1998, it was really getting tough on me at home, so I said, "Let me come and stay with you, and I'll support all the other children in my mother's house. We'll see how it works out." But I was soon tearing myself in two pieces because every day after work I'd stop at my mother's house before driving to his home. He was insisting that he also needed me. I got very tired.

'When he said he really didn't want to see the other kids in his house, I had a hard choice to make. I asked myself, "Do I want to live this way for the rest of my life?" I thought if he's treating the others like this now, maybe at some point he'll end up treating his stepson, Bosco, like that. I was probably being unfair because he's not the type of person who cares only for his own kid, Betty. Bosco's one of the reasons he wanted to stick with us up till now.

'The thing that made me decide to move on was that he didn't understand why I was working at TASO. He said, "I can open up a job for you paying three times that." But it's not the money. I have to feel I have done something useful to be at peace with my conscience. He never appreciated that.'

Sophia isn't alone in encountering resistance from her man.

'I used to think he behaved the way he did because he's white,' she says. 'but two of the ladies who clean the TASO offices recently told me their stories. Molly and her partner both have AIDS. He has his own children and she has her own children from her first husband. His children stay with them but he won't let her bring hers into their house so they have to stay at her parents' place.

'And the other lady, Phoebe, says her husband won't let her relatives come to their house either. She doesn't have any children but she has to bring up his. So I think women are just more willing to take on relatives than men.'

Some women hesitate to take in their relatives' orphans because they fear that their husband will abuse them. It's easier to absorb children from his side of the family because the taboo of incest inhibits sexual abuse. 'In our culture,' explains Sophia, 'children from the wife's side can easily become co-wives, because the husband doesn't have a blood relationship with them'.

TASO has started a project for their clients' orphans. They identify the best students and pay their fees at boarding schools. They're paying a million shillings (about £400) a year per child for 232 children to get a good education.

'We don't think it's an extravagant strategy,' says Sophia. 'because it means the least time in abusive foster families where they do all the donkey work and don't have time to study'.

The programme's director, Reverend Benjamin Mpomba-Kakonge tells foster parents who are jealous that the orphan is being singled out for assistance, 'Look, if I take this child from your home, I'm lessening the burden on you.' He reminds them of the numbers of AIDS orphans and the fact that many have sent all their own children to school before the orphan.

Potential scholars sit an exam and a committee of people from TASO visits clients' homes, without an appointment, to establish how poor they are, how many children they have and how the orphan is treated. They then decide who gets the opportunity.

'We know we can only help so many orphans,' says Rev Mpomba-Kakonge. 'and we want our programme to have an impact. We want to produce a doctor. Or, for those who have gone to vocational schools, we want them to have skills that are marketable like carpentry.'

Rose spends a lot of her time at the TASO head office. She's 21, pretty and bright, but sad. She maintains eye contact with people as if she needs to keep checking that she's being accepted. She lost her parents to AIDS in the 1980s when the stigma around the disease was much worse than it is now, and was cast out by her relatives.

Rose is one of TASO's stars because she's made it to Makerere University in Kampala, Uganda's best university. TASO pays the fees. She works hard and is painfully grateful. She shows it by opening and sorting Sophia's mail every day.

She is a petite girl with big fearful eyes.

'I'm an orphan', she says, softly. 'My father died and then my mother checked her blood and found out she was HIV-positive in 1985. I was six then. She joined TASO, which had just begun. It had a scheme, which used to pay school fees for kids who performed well in school. They took me on.

'I was born to Mr Mutembeya, but I never knew him and then he died. My mother married another man and we joined his family. They separated and I had to go with her and take care of her because she was sick by then. She didn't really talk to me about it. I think her problem was me. Whenever she was in pain, she'd worry, "Who will take care of my daughter?"

'It was in the late '80s and AIDS made her a social reject. My mother's family abandoned her. All my friends ran away because they thought we would infect them. We stuck together alone. I was taking care of her, however young I was. TASO became my family.

'I feel angry that our real family ran away. Maybe it's affected me psychologically. I still visit them occasionally, when I have time off school, but I still have what they did in my mind.

'I was twelve when my mum died in 1992. I'd just completed primary school. I was staying with an uncle but he didn't want me ... ' Rose's chin trembles. 'I was staying with my mum's brother, but they never liked me. OK, they couldn't show it directly but they would do some peculiar things to show you that you don't belong here.

'It's difficult talking about these painful things, but I know if you keep talking about it, you will cease to have that pain in your heart.'

TASO gave Rose the chance to go to boarding school.

'It was hard to make friends at school because everyone said, "That girl's mother died of AIDS." They wouldn't hug me.' Rose's voice trails off to a whisper. 'I didn't like it but what could I do? If people came to me, I'd welcome them, and those who didn't … I had to give up and study. When I was unhappy, I'd work harder. I got good grades. If you come up as a poor girl, what else can you do? You just have to take every opportunity. I'm always ready to learn. My mum wanted me to be educated, so that I will become a somebody, somehow, somewhere in the future.'

TASO have the names of 200,000 children like Rose on their books. They have 259 staff at seven branches.

'To begin with, we were just paying school fees,' says Sophia. 'but now we're trying to improve how we communicate with children. We used to just see the child as part of a family, "Your parents are sick so you have to do this to help them." But now, we're talking to the children separately, as children, and we're trying to start looking after them before their mothers die.'

People find it difficult to tell their children that they're HIV-positive. Many don't. TASO are involved in a project to train parents to write a 'memory book' for their children. It's like a scrapbook, full of family photos. The parent writes about where she came from, her lineage and describes herself. She includes her dreams for the child. She might also mention how she got, or suspect she got, infected, to try to deal with the issue of blame. The book's aim is to help the child build an identity. When the parent dies it may be the only evidence of where they came from. It's better for the child if the parent writes it with him because he'll understand more. But it's not easy. Many parents write a memory book and leave it with a friend to give to their children after they die.

The Memory Book Project is run jointly by TASO, Save the Children and another Ugandan NGO called the National Community of Women Living with HIV/AIDS (NACWOLA). Beatrice Were, who runs the latter, has been HIV-positive for eight years. She knows how hard it is to write a memory book. She has two children and is half way through her first one for her older child. It takes time to gather all the information you need from far-flung relatives and it costs money to have family photos printed to make it beautiful. Only a fifth of the 150 women trained to make memory books in

NACWOLA's recent pilot project in Kampala had actually completed one a few months later.

When TASO started, people came needing material help and medical care because they were already sick with AIDS. Some expected a job or handouts. Others came hoping for a longer life.

To encourage people to benefit from TASO's counselling services, the staff made it compulsory. If you wanted pills, you had to talk your worries through first. Initially, clients didn't mind this, but once they started coping again, some would actually invent problems to discuss. So TASO stopped forcing counselling on people. But still, by 1999, more people were coming for counselling than for medicine. In the late 1990s, more Ugandans started getting tested for HIV, so many came to TASO for counselling while still healthy. Knowing that you are HIV-positive is traumatic, but it allows time to prepare for your children's future, and possibly write a memory book.

Sophia thinks that more Ugandans are going for the HIV test because the society is getting used to the disease.

> 'Everyone knows people who aren't immoral, but are still infected. Like my sister. She was one of the most faithful wives, but she still got infected. Most AIDS orphans would say the same thing about their mothers. I think HIV's been demystified. And things definitely improved when the government came out in 1986 and said, "Hey, we have a problem here. We have HIV."'

It's easy to like Sophia's kids. On a Saturday morning, four of them – Stanley, Sandy, Bosco and Betty – are lounging around at home. Sandy and Bosco play cards games, while a video, *The Lion King II,* plays in the background. Bosco knows every line of the script.

Sandy is a tall and confident teenager. He's 17 and in his last year of school and wants to study mass communications or maybe law afterwards. Sophia says, 'Sandy doesn't fear anything. He's not ashamed to talk about his parents having died of AIDS.' He has an easy charm. He's slender and handsome. He's happy to show a visitor a poem he's written for Sophia. Each stanza starts with a capital letter, which spells out 'MOTHER' down the page. It ends, 'I'm really grateful.' It's easy to see why she adopted him.

Sandy picks up a pen to draw his family tree. He explains who's who in his big family, as he sketches rows of wives and children under his father's name. He can't remember the names of three of the wives so he puts Xs for them, but he vaguely remembers their children at their father's funeral. He adds everybody's tribe's name and puts asterisks by 15 of the children's names to show which ones stay in touch with each other.

Stanley, by contrast, is shy. He's 20 and studying for a degree in computing. It's impossible to guess what he's thinking.

When Sandy and Stanley's father was dying, he proposed that seven of his children, especially his three heirs – Sandy, Stanley and Samuel, all the eldest sons of different wives – should go to live in the UK. But when he died, their father's brother, a prominent politician, overruled the idea. The boys were livid. But now, as Sandy observes, 'There's no point being angry for ever.' Plus the man pays for their education.

Sandy writes 'destitute' next to the twins' and their brother Ssalongo's names. He describes the twins as 'sluts, whores'. He says that they had everything the others had, but they chose to go out dancing, drinking and having sex.

Little Bosco, who's ten, is slightly titillated by the older children's behaviour. 'One of the twins is pregnant,' he announces. 'and Sadic's been suspended from school … and Ssalongo took someone's eye out in a fight'.

Betty is the baby. She's seven and has cute plaits that stick out at interesting angles. She's shy initially but is soon parading through the living room in just her knickers, giggling. She changes her clothes three times in two hours and finally selects a pinafore dress over a Barbie T-shirt. Her big brothers love her. She's the only one with two living parents.

When there are just four kids there, Sophia's house isn't too crowded. When all ten are at home, however, it gets quite frantic. Sophia's side of the family isn't small either. Apart from Susan, Sophia has another four sisters. Some of Sophia's relatives live in the compound with her, her elderly mother and a pack of constantly scrapping yellow dogs.

One Saturday afternoon, Sophia is tied up with a TASO meeting so asks John, a driver employed by TASO, to take the kids to Sharrot's school for a special Open Day. Sharrot's siblings get smartened up and cram into the back of John's four-by-four. The school is some way out of Kampala and on the way Sandy chattily points out the cemetery where all the family members are buried. John deftly dodges yawning potholes.

The children are dropped off at the bottom of the driveway up to Sharrot's imposing private girls' school. Soldiers with machine guns frisk visitors. There's serious security because the First Lady, Janet Museveni, is the Guest of Honour for the official opening of a new campus. The impressive building has sprung up in the last three months. There's a row of seven brand new computers in one of the dusty new classrooms.

Rows of VIPs and parents sit under canopies. The women wear brightly coloured dresses with gravity-defying, big puffy shoulders. Their hair is exquisitely coiffured with extensions and sculpted curls stuck in place. The men wear suits. It's a hot afternoon and the speeches have already been going for two hours. Sandy joins the audience of well-heeled parents. Betty wriggles on his lap. He lovingly readjusts the tangled straps of her pinafore dress.

Coke bottles litter the ground. Girls in uniforms quietly collect them as the speeches go on. They huddle, eye up Sandy, and whisper behind their hands, while the First Lady gives a rousing speech about these girls being a part of The New Uganda because they're strong women and proud Africans. She also talks about all the millions of kids in the developing world who are missing out on school.

Mrs Museveni started an NGO, Uganda Women's Effort to Save Orphans (UWESO) in 1986, to care for orphans of the civil war that scorched Uganda in the early 1980s. Initially the charity provided food and blankets. Later, AIDS orphans began to outnumber war orphans. UWESO provided school fees for them until they became frustrated that their efforts were high cost and low impact in that they weren't reaching many children. In 1994, they changed their approach and now provide training and $100 in credit for female guardians to establish small businesses. In 2000, they had about 4,000 such entrepreneurs. Indirectly, an estimated 100,000 orphans across 35 districts were benefiting.

Finally the speeches end and a cake is cut. A tinny rendition of 'Congratulations and celebrations' is piped over the speakers. It has been impossible to spot Sharrot until she emerges out of the crowd of girls in blue ties and white knee socks. She's delighted that her family has turned up to support her, but a bossy prefect shoos her back towards the school group. They're not released again. VIPs, soldiers and parents drift away.

Watching Sophia's children on this outing is heart-warming. Sandy keeps an eye out for Bosco, who's wandered off bored, and stops Betty falling off a balcony. She hangs round his neck. There are no quarrels all day. When posing for a photo the older boys put their arms around the younger two. It isn't forced. There's real fondness.

The scale of the orphans' loss is huge. Sandy, for instance, has lost his father, his mother and his baby brother. But he now lives with his aunt, who is sensitive and caring. His education to tertiary level is assured. He has social skills. He may carry sorrow, but he's doing all right.

On the other hand, the twins are in crisis. They have lost their father and their mother. Their brother is in prison. They're only 16, but they've dropped out of school and are having risky sex for money.

This one family has seen more than its share of tragedy, but somehow, it holds together, more or less. The surviving children have enough to eat and the opportunity to go to school. Some have coped. Others have not. Fifteen are still in contact with each other and gain some sort of support from belonging to a group of people who shared a father. They're lucky in that their extended family is able and willing to provide for them, but they must, at times, feel like a burden to Sophia and the uncle who pays for their schooling, whether they're reminded of this 'debt' regularly, occasionally or not at all.

As Uganda's AIDS epidemic matures, a child who lives with two parents is now the exception. The need for people like Sophia, prepared to provide love and shelter to children besides her own, grows daily more acute. For Sophia, it has entailed considerable sacrifices. But charity has its rewards, too. Sophia's kids know she isn't obliged to be there for them, so they're very appreciative. It might not be the family Sophia planned, but it is a loving, extended one.

3
Strangers Step In

The Tale of Two Foster Parents, South Africa

'The South African Child Welfare system exists for the welfare of its employees. They're power-crazed, inefficient and utterly crass. If someone told me they had proof that South Africa is actually practising an unofficial policy of infanticide, it wouldn't surprise me at all.' These are the words of Lawrence Smith, a professor of English literature. He and his wife, Fiona saw television coverage of the AIDS orphan crisis and decided they wanted to help. They offered to take an HIV-positive child into their home. Social workers made it nearly impossible.

Child Welfare is the generic name given to the 169 autonomous branches affiliated to a national organisation, the South African National Council for Child and Family Welfare. They are a non-governmental organisation (NGO) but their social workers' salaries are heavily subsidised by the state. About 90 per cent of their work is statutory: finding homes for the abused and abandoned children who find themselves in 'the system'.

In rich countries, with well-developed child welfare infrastructure, adoption is considered to be the best option for orphans because it offers security by permanently transferring legal guardianship to the new parents. Fostering is seen as a short-term fix, usually with a view to returning the child to its parents or whilst finding adoptive parents.

Formal fostering and adoption will only ever be able to help small numbers of AIDS orphans in Africa. Fostering is usually done informally by relatives. For many children, this provides a happy and permanent solution, unhindered by bureaucracy. Where state welfare systems are minimal or non-existent, few people worry about legal niceties.

In 2000, South African Welfare Minister Zola Skweyiya estimated that about a third of the country's 250,000 AIDS orphans were in foster care, and almost two-thirds were being cared for by their families or communities. Perhaps 0.25 per cent were in orphanages and 0.1 per cent had been formally adopted.

The state must step in when children have fallen through the safety net that families and communities usually provide. Abandoned babies epitomise this group, and their numbers have increased sharply. In one year (1998–99), social workers at the South African National Council for Child and Family Welfare saw the number of foundlings they dealt with more than double. By 2000, an estimated 3,000 children were being abandoned annually. AIDS is probably to blame. In Africa, HIV-positive mothers receive little, if any, counselling. They assume that they are going to die soon and that their baby will automatically be infected.

All children born to infected mothers initially test positive for HIV, because their mothers' antibodies are present in their blood. However, the majority of them lose these antibodies, become HIV-negative and go on to live healthy lives. The Elisa HIV antibody test to confirm a child's HIV status can be done after 15–18 months. There are various other tests, which can be done from two weeks, which identify the virus itself or particles of the virus, but all are prohibitively expensive for routine use. In sub-Saharan Africa, about a third of the children born to HIV-positive mothers will become infected *in utero*, during labour or via breast milk. Many die within two years; few live beyond five. With good basic care, this number can be increased.

Jenny was abandoned at five weeks old on someone's doorstep. The police took her to a hospital where she tested HIV-positive. Since Fiona and Lawrence took her in, she has tested HIV-negative. She's now a healthy, chubby baby, asleep in the middle of their double bed.

Fiona is 39. Lawrence is 55. They have been married for seven and a half years and have no children of their own. They have both been married before. Fiona lost three babies in two miscarriages in her previous marriage. They both stress that infertility is not their reason for fostering Jenny.

Lawrence says, 'I never wanted children once I realised I couldn't have them. This isn't having a child in that kind of way. It's a response to a social need. In September 1999, we kept seeing news programmes about AIDS orphans. They were talking about up to two million AIDS orphans in South Africa. We looked at one another and said, "Surely not. All these little kids in institutions. If we can only help one ..."'

Fiona continues, 'I'm one of those people who go through life thinking if every motorist stopped, and let one person through, you'd never have a traffic jam. I feel the same way about this. OK, we don't have much money, and no experience whatsoever, but we thought we could love a child and make it feel secure and special.'

Fiona's only half joking when she describes how uninterested in children she has been, until now.

'From the age of twelve, I said I wouldn't have any. My friends used to keep theirs away from me, because I can't stand them. I'd tell them I'm allergic to them. I break out in hives!

'I don't know what's the greatest shock for people: me getting a baby, an HIV baby or a black baby. I'm not sure. I think it's probably me with a baby. When I phoned my mum, who's an unflappable, retired midwife, and said, "We're thinking about looking after an HIV baby", she said, "I'm in shock", and put the phone down. To her credit, she phoned back 20 minutes later and said it was wonderful.

'Yes, I'm 40 next week, broody and all the rest of it, but this isn't a substitute for our own child. The way I feel about Jenny is still a shock for me. It was instant. And it's Jenny. It's not just any child. I don't want another one. We love *her*. She's my baby. She's my child. I can't explain it ...'

Fiona looks gaunt and anxious talking about the events of the last few months. Her ribs show through the satin slip of a dress she wears around the house on a steamy, hot afternoon. Lawrence looks less fragile. He's a grey-haired academic, originally from Yorkshire in England. He came to South Africa in 1972. Their home is unfussy. It has been tidied, probably for the arrival of Fiona's mother tomorrow. She's coming to visit her first grandchild for the first time. Known for her excellent malapropisms, she's been calling Jenny, 'Fiona's VIP baby' rather than an HIV baby.

Fiona made history in 1950 by being South Africa's first exported baby.

'I was born in Cape Town and was sent to South West Africa, which is now Namibia. This wasn't official policy. They weren't meant to be sending children over borders. But they tried saying

"No" to my dad, and you didn't say "No" to him because then he'd say, "Now I *really* want one." He already had two grown-up kids and wasn't sure he wanted another until they tried to obstruct. My mother had lost five babies. She was desperate to have one.

'My records are still sealed. That was post-adoption procedure in those days. They're sealed till 2060, although I've met everyone involved because someone left my birth certificate lying around, and my adoptive mother saw the birth mother's name. And she tracked this woman down, I think probably illegally, by getting into computers or something. But she did it, and encouraged me to meet my biological mother. I had to go to America to meet her and I wasn't particularly keen. It was a total disaster and she subsequently died. She was 15 when she had me. I've always known I was adopted. I can't remember ever *not* knowing.'

Fiona left school at 16 and worked as a secretary in the insurance business. She then ran an architect's office. Her mother introduced her to Lawrence and they were married six weeks later. She enrolled as a mature student at the university where he lectured and later taught there too.

She's acutely aware of South Africans' risk of contracting AIDS. When her well-heeled, post-apartheid generation students declare 'I won't get AIDS', she tells them that she was car-jacked on campus and raped.

While Jenny is sleeping, Fiona chain-smokes on the veranda. She repeatedly denies smoking near the baby and often says, 'We've nothing to hide.' Contact with Child Welfare has made them paranoid. Although they have been screened by social workers, the paperwork's completed and a court order has placed Jenny with them on a fostering basis, they still worry that, without warning or explanation, Jenny might be whisked away. It has already happened once.

When Jenny had been with them for a week, she was removed and sent back to a children's home. After three weeks of frantic phone calls, legal threats and stress, she was returned to them. The social workers clearly did not have a fundamental objection to the Smiths looking after children, because during those three traumatic weeks, they offered them a different baby.

Fiona says, 'When they took her away, they said, "There's a baby at this hospital. Would you be interested in it?" I said, "We'd like *our* baby back. Why can't we have her back?"'

For the Smiths, the process of getting a child started with a visit to their local Child Welfare office.

'Once we'd decided to foster a baby, we assumed that the procedures would be gone through, in a serious but not protracted way', says Lawrence. 'We assumed that if there's a national crisis of abandoned and orphaned children, there would be systems to deal with it. But that's not what we found.

'When we went to see Child Welfare, we said we'd heard the figure of 1–2 million AIDS orphans. "Oh, not here", cries this social worker.'

Fiona takes up the story, 'She told us, "This isn't really a problem, because the black community is now *owning* the problem. There are no abandoned babies at the moment."'

Lawrence and Fiona don't believe there was no problem of abandoned babies in their area. 'What they mean is there may not be a problem in their geographical jurisdiction', says Lawrence. 'It's very territorial. We've found they work within their own little fiefdoms.'

The director of the branch of Child Welfare Lawrence and Fiona went to says,

'It goes in waves. At the moment there are only two kids in our shelter and they're there because they're HIV-positive. We're not overwhelmed. A television programme will show all these HIV-positive children languishing in children's homes. After it, we'll get lots of requests and we say we don't have any at the moment.'

A couple seeking a baby in one part of the country will not be introduced to a child needing a family in another part of the country.

Fiona and Lawrence were impatient.

'We arrived for our first appointment with Child Welfare,' says Fiona, 'and got a 20-minute history lesson about their organisation and a long story about a Christmas party they were planning for some children. We just wanted to say, "Look, where are the forms? Interview us. Let's get this moving."'

Lawrence continues, 'They asked the obvious questions like, "Are you wanting to foster or adopt?" We said we didn't want a full-blown AIDS baby right away because we weren't sure what it's like having children in the first place. Our initial plan was to take an HIV baby, which would be re-tested at 15 months. And then, if she were positive we would keep her for the duration and if she were negative, we'd rethink.'

Fiona adds, 'I told them, "It's 6 October and we're ready. We've spoken to people in the field. We've bought a few things like bottles and nappies. We don't know much about HIV but we're two intelligent and, I think, responsible people. We've both finished work, me because the course I was teaching had ended and Lawrence for three months' leave, which means we'll both be at home for the next three months."

'We were put on hold. It was three weeks before anybody contacted us. First they said it would take six weeks. Then three months. At that initial meeting they said we'd have a home visit by a social worker within a week or two. After three weeks, I phoned and asked what was happening. I think I was labelled as being pushy.

'It got worse. They labelled us "too intense" because we'd gone out and bought a baby bath. I didn't want to be like my parents who got me and were totally unprepared.'

Lawrence and Fiona think they were seen as trouble-makers because they got ready too quickly and because they hassled staff to move faster than their system permitted.

Finally, after more delays, Fiona and Lawrence received a half-hour screening visit by two women from Child Welfare. 'Do you have a full-time maid?' they asked Fiona.

'No,' she replied, 'I'm married to a British socialist. And in any case, what's that got to do with it? I'll be looking after the child, with Lawrence. We're going to be hands on.'

The social workers seemed to be concerned about cross-cultural families. Fiona told them,

'Look, we've got the university crèche directly opposite our home, which is multiracial.' She continues, 'I'd already booked the child in and I'd gone to see the Professor of Zulu to work out a nice Zulu name for this child. I'd also just taught a six-month course on Zulu traditions comparing them with Ancient Roman and Greek rituals. Look, we're not going to slaughter a goat if she marries, and dance around with *assegais* [spears] as she leaves our home. No, we're not. I'm Eurocentric. Sorry. But I probably know more about Zulu initiation rites than the average person on the street and she'll be bilingual. I speak enough Zulu.'

She gets exasperated. 'Lawrence is English. I'm South African. She's a Zulu. We'll figure it out. But what really irritated me was the fact that if she was HIV-positive, which she was when we got her, and dead by two, what the hell does it matter? Let's worry about that later. She's a little baby and she needs assistance now.'

Around the world, many people view transracial adoption with suspicion because the child may grow up culturally confused. South Africa, where race colours every interaction, is no exception. South African whites who've adopted black children sometimes get pressure from both sides; whites saying, 'Why? This isn't your child' and blacks saying, 'Why are you stealing our children?'

Abandoned babies present a problem for South African social workers. No one knows if a black foundling is a Zulu, a Xhosa or what. Such babies languish in hospitals and children's homes while their legal status is sorted out. Meanwhile, they are exposed to a hotchpotch of cultural influences.

For orphanage staff trying to place children as quickly as possible, culture is a minor consideration, and white people who have adopted black children from orphanages find the prejudices of those who oppose transracial adoption in all circumstances frustrating. They feel it does not matter. Children should not be in institutions.

'By the time we got to see the director of this branch on 18 December, we'd done everything the system required of us', recollects Fiona. 'They told us to have this done. We do it. Then there's something else. We do it. And much of their information was wrong. We were told we had to go on a HIV/AIDS course. It didn't exist. Then we were told we had to go to the local hospice for bereavement counselling for when the child dies. We'd also gone to see the crack HIV paediatrician at a local hospital.'

This doctor recollects Lawrence and Fionas' visit. He's concerned that people are moved by sensational television coverage of AIDS orphans. Some rush forward wanting to foster or adopt children or open an orphanage without fully considering the implications. He also feels that the necessary support systems to help new foster parents are lacking.

Frustrated with the delays, Lawrence and Fiona side-stepped Child Welfare and unofficially became 'host parents' for Jenny, a child from Blossom Children's Home, a home and hospice for HIV-positive children. A host parent is a volunteer who regularly takes a child out from an orphanage, for a day or a weekend at a time.

Jenny seemed to be at death's door when they got her.

'We received Jenny on 26 November because Fiona had made contact with Jean who runs Blossom Children's Home', says Lawrence. 'During a phone call, Jean said that she was very worried about a particular child, Jenny, because she was so ill. She was scared that if Jenny stayed there over the weekend of 26–28 November, she might die. We said, "OK, we'll take her." After the weekend, we said, "Look, she's thriving. Can we keep her?"'

Fiona picks up the story, 'The assumption was she was HIV-positive. She looked awful. She had a drip in her head. But within five days, she went from drinking under 100 to 650 millilitres a day. If you have 40 babies, like they do at Blossom Children's Home, you don't have time to constantly feed and play with them. That's all we did for the week she was here.'

Lawrence continues, 'Somehow the Child Welfare people who'd placed Jenny at Blossom Children's Home, a different branch to the one we'd been dealing with, learnt that we were hosting her. And because our paperwork wasn't complete, they freaked. The truth is that the social worker had messed up and she was trying to cover her tracks.'

There is no legal definition of abandonment or time limit before a child can be declared abandoned. It can take months to sort out. Staff from several agencies must be involved to obtain a birth certificate, get a medical report done and try to trace the mother. Officials in different towns require different levels of proof. Some, for instance, require the abandoned child's photograph to have been advertised in a local paper. The more time lapses, the less likely that the child will be reunited with her family.

'Jenny's social worker had lost her photo,' says Fiona, 'so had failed to put it in the press. She started threatening us, "We've found the mother and we're doing DNA testing." This was absolute garbage.

'The long and the short of it was that Jenny had to go back to Blossom Children's Home because of a lack of paper', says Lawrence. 'I got one of our three referees, a lawyer, to intervene on our behalf, to see if she couldn't stay here pending the paperwork being completed.'

'So she wouldn't die', says Fiona quietly. 'There was chicken pox at Blossom Children's Home and if she'd got it she would have died. She was that fragile.'

Lawrence continues, 'Our lawyer friend had a chilling conversation with Jenny's social worker in which she said, "No, according to the rules, Jenny has to go back to Blossom Children's Home." And he said, "I understand her health is at risk and she might die." "Even if she dies", said the social worker. He was appalled.'

So after a week with Lawrence and Fiona, Jenny went back to Blossom Children's Home. Her new parents grieved for her. They couldn't understand what was happening.

'That last morning, when I was feeding her, I was trying not to cry aloud so she wouldn't be affected by it. But inside I was howling. I had bonded with her instantly. Lawrence had dropped me off at Blossom Children's Home and gone off to collect something. Jean said, "Here's your daughter. She's hungry. Feed her", and I said, "Oh, OK." Lawrence came back two hours later and I was just holding her ...'

'I walked into this room and my wife was a changed woman. She had this kind of glow of commitment. It was wonderful to see.'

It took three weeks to straighten out the paperwork and get Jenny back.

'I've lost about ten kilos since we started this', says Fiona. 'I was haggard. The worst thing was feeling like we'd let her down.'

Meanwhile, staff at Fiona and Lawrences' branch of Child Welfare were still going through the process to select or reject them as foster parents. There were further delays, lies and nastiness. Finally, a state social worker commissioned a social worker from a different agency to screen them.

Lawrence says, 'Assuming the system's intended to work for the welfare of the children, and not the apparatchiks who are employed by it, it doesn't seem to be working.'

'Different people tell you different things,' says Fiona. 'and sometimes the same person tells you different things on different days. At one point, I hadn't heard anything for a fortnight, so I rang and asked, "What's the story?" and the social worker said, "I'm thinking that the next baby is yours." I phoned Lawrence. I phoned my mum. I'm saying, "The baby's coming. Do you think it'll be a boy?" And then later, they say, "Oh no, she never said that to you." Why would I lie about something like that? Explain it to me, because I don't understand.'

When Jenny was returned to Blossom Children's Home, Fiona was beside herself. She spent days on the phone, trying to get the Child Welfare staff to contact their referees. The staff would claim to have faxed forms out, but referees wouldn't receive them. In the end, one out of three referees was contacted. Two days before the court case, at which Jenny's transfer to Fiona and Lawrence as a place of safety was meant to be approved, the social worker who'd originally placed Jenny at Blossom Children's Home called for an indefinite adjournment. Fiona believes she hadn't got the paperwork together. Child Welfare held an emergency meeting on Christmas Eve to discuss their case.

Fiona continues the saga, 'They didn't phone us. Lawrence phoned them and came running, saying, "Get dressed, we're going to pick her up." And I was saying, "Thank you so much. I love you so much for getting my baby back." And he said, "Shut up. Get in the car. We're going."' Fiona laughs at the memory.

They were now registered as a place of safety. This is meant to be a six-week stop-gap until a longer-term foster placement can be found for a child. It took another two months before they officially became her foster parents.

'We brought back the most insecure baby. She didn't sleep till Christmas Day. She went 18 hours without sleep. There's no doubt that she knew me instantly. I picked her up and she just went into my neck like a little monkey. Within a few days, it was as though she'd never gone. I still wake up in shock thinking, "This is unreal."'

'I don't know whether our experiences are typical', admits Lawrence. 'All we know is the story we have to tell. But look at it this way, if it's going to take you three months to screen potential parents, they're not going to get the children out of the system. Why is it so inefficient? Why is there not more funding? There's funding for official cars for provincial politicians.'

Lawrence and Fiona's experience makes little sense. People who volunteer to care for needy children should be better managed. When a selection process questions people's suitability to be parents, clients need to be treated tactfully. Weeks later, Fiona and Lawrence are still smarting from being labelled 'too intense' and not told why.

Obviously there is no policy of infanticide in South Africa. Lawrence and Fiona are clearly wrong on this count. But neither are children smoothly placed in loving homes.

Petro Brink, a private adoption expert, offers a better explanation for Fiona and Lawrences' experiences. She compares social workers to the police. Both are badly paid, demotivated and dehumanised by constant contact with victims of violence or abuse. Without support, they burn out. Then if they don't leave the job, they are at risk of crossing a line, over which they stop caring. Some become sullen and obstructive. Some even start to abuse the children in their care. Brutalised policemen too often end up beating up suspects or their own wives. Social workers, especially those who have specialised in child abuse, can become more subtly brutalised. Without good supervision, the power over other people's lives can corrupt them and they may consequently 'abuse' people like Fiona and Lawrence.

Every day, South African social workers are exposed to a bottomless pit of human need, most of it related to poverty. They don't have the resources to put things right. Some social workers' officious manner may stem from feelings of powerlessness. The job is stressful and there are few opportunities for promotion. Young, inexperienced social workers replace those who leave to seek better pay and job security as bank clerks or secretaries. Turnover is rapid.

There are, of course, many excellent Child Welfare staff, but the system gives them little support. Supervision is minimal, so inefficiency and incompetence are widespread. Everyone criticises social workers. Like the police, they feel victimised and defensive.

The current criteria for selecting parents are negative. The system works by looking for people's flaws, instead of looking for what positive things people are offering.

Social workers at the Child Welfare office, which dealt with the Smiths, have an average of 40 cases at any one time. They are counselling women who want to give up their babies, investigating and placing abandoned children and arranging adoptions with families, the latter usually for step-parents or grandmothers who want to formalise their relationship with a child they're already caring for. The Special Needs Co-ordinator (who places HIV-positive and disabled children) has about 25 HIV-positive children to place, a similar number of foster parents, and will be screening about ten more potential parents at the same time.

It took seven weeks from the time Fiona and Lawrence offered themselves as parents to the day they got Jenny and then a further three months before they were officially her foster parents. This felt like an eternity. Having no knowledge of the convoluted system, Fiona and Lawrence could not fathom why it was taking so long, and the social workers they dealt with made no attempt to explain.

People who have made the big decision to take in a child, will inevitably arrive all fired up to have one immediately. A supervisor at the Child Welfare explains that it's very difficult to tell potential parents how long the process will take. Also, potential parents usually arrive with very specific age and gender requests. They want a child old enough to go into a crèche while they work or a new-born that they can claim is their own to avoid the stigma of infertility.

The rules need to be clarified and simplified. Not all potential parents will be as assertive as the Smiths. Some may be more easily put off, when they encounter the delays, errors and evasions that stem from an overloaded system.

Even though Lawrence and Fiona had 'won' Jenny back, after weeks of fighting the system, her future with them remained uncertain for a while.

Lawrence was saying, 'We don't know whether we'll eventually adopt her. Fiona's adoptive father died when she was seven. It was a very traumatic experience for her and I'd hate to do that to Jenny.

'There's also the slight problem that the university stops our employment at 60, which is why we thought in terms of a terminally ill child when we went into this. I don't want Jenny to be in tough straits as well as us, so we're going to have to take some time thinking it through. The important thing is to give her what we can now.'

At the same time, Fiona was saying, 'I knew I would look after her, nurse her and love her. She's a little helpless thing. I knew I would care for her, like I would a cat. But I never thought I'd feel like this about her. Not in a billion years. Lawrence says he's seen a new ... What was it you said that was so sweet?'

'I just watched you doing what you were doing with a kind of awe. You were ...'

Fiona remembers, 'You said, "I thought I knew you but I didn't have any idea of this love. I see people and they say you are lit up from within. Yes, you look tired but all the tension is gone from your face." Lawrence doesn't compliment me that often!' She smiles.

Fiona gets out a journal she has started for Jenny. She wants Jenny to continue writing it as soon as she's able. It is full of photos of Jenny from Day One with them. It shows the rapid progress from skinny, sick child to well-fed, happier child. Over the pictures, there are captions written in a computer's childish font. It is written as if from Jenny's perspective, with lots of exclamation marks.

Most of Lawrence's colleagues have teenage children. He says,

'They look at me with new eyes because I've never had children. I think it's taken some of them aback. But they're terribly excited about it. I think it's intrigued some people because I'm not politically correct. I don't buy the PC rubbish some academics come out with.'

Fiona interjects, 'Yes, funny how your street cred goes up!'

The catalyst for Lawrence and Fionas' decision to foster a child was media coverage of the numbers of AIDS orphans needing homes. Without that, they probably would never have considered taking on a child. They asked for a short-term, intense commitment – an HIV-positive child. Instead they fostered Jenny, a healthy baby. The system allows them two years to decide what to do next, because a foster child's situation is reviewed every two years. This story has a rare happy ending because within a year, they had officially adopted her. Even in their earlier indecision, it had seemed unlikely that they would be able to give her up, especially having experienced the agonies of a three-week, forced separation.

Fiona says with relish, 'I wasn't born to be a mother. I was born to be *her* mother. There is a link between this child and me. I believe in reincarnation and I know Lawrence and I were somehow linked before, and Jenny and I definitely were.'

'I don't see things in these mystical terms,' says Lawrence, 'but she's lovely to have around'.

Section II

Projects

4
Childcare by Committee

A Social Worker's Story, Pietermaritzburg, South Africa

Bongi Zengele is a rarity: a *cheerful* South African social worker. She works in Pietermaritzburg, the second biggest town after Durban in South Africa's KwaZulu-Natal province. The architecture and genteel shops in the centre look prosperously English, but the shacks on the edge of town remind one how poor most of the town's inhabitants are. Unlike many in her demoralised profession, Bongi remains jovial and self-motivated. She wears big, flowing dresses and her bespectacled eyes twinkle when she laughs.

South Africa's child welfare system is caught between two worlds. Under apartheid a formal fostering and adoption system, imitating British and American practices, was developed for needy children amongst the country's five million whites. Almost no such services were available to other races and transracial adoptions were banned.

Since the first democratic elections in 1994, the system has been in flux. Services are now, in theory at least, available to 42 million South Africans. Even without AIDS, the system would not be able to cope. Childcare legislation is being reviewed; more flexible, cheaper and quicker ways of caring are sought. But the process is fraught with practical and ethical problems.

Many South African social workers are stressed by all the changes. They did a four-year degree, which prepared them to do 'case work' identifying child abuse, counselling individuals, processing the statutory requirements for fostering and adoption placements and so on. But now the government says they must shift from the old, First World-style services to a more developmental approach. There's a lot of woolly discussion of what this means, but in practice it's about encouraging poor people to help themselves and not wait for welfare grants and services that simply aren't going to materialise. In the context of the AIDS epidemic, development work is about spreading welfare services thinner (cutting down on complicated, time-consuming work like adoptions) in order to reach more orphans, and getting communities to take care of children so they're kept out of costly orphanages.

College courses are changing to accommodate the new approach, but not fast enough. Many graduates rapidly leave the profession for less stressful, better-paid jobs, or emigrate. Social workers often feel overwhelmed by the numbers of children needing their help and are ill-equipped to help them. Some have tried to resist change because they resent what they see as a lowering of standards.

Bongi personifies the shift. She was educated at the prestigious University of the Witwatersrand in Johannesburg, graduating in 1993, a year before apartheid ended. For a few years she did old-style social work: finding foster and adoptive parents for orphaned and abandoned children. But then she switched to working for a project that sets up committees of volunteers who keep an eye out for needy children in their communities. The work requires a completely different mindset.

Bongi, who's now 35, has cared for children all her life, having brought up her five sisters from the age of eight. She has also recently inherited two children from relatives.

The incident that inspired her to train to be a social worker happened in 1988, when the KwaZulu and Natal region was consumed by political violence. During the 1980s and 1990s, over 12,000 people died in the undeclared war between the African National Congress (ANC) and the Inkatha Freedom Party (IFP). The violence eased after South Africa's first democratic election in 1994, but it didn't stop. In the Edendale Valley where Bongi was doing volunteer church work, whole families were massacred. One night, an elderly couple was shot dead. The killers thought they'd finished everyone in the house, but later Bongi found a four-year-old grandson hiding under a bed.

'I came from the township of Claremont,' she says, 'A community of activists and outspoken youths. At school, we were getting into all sorts of political involvements … I wanted to change the world.' She hoots with laughter.

'But the first year of my degree seemed completely out of my context. It was all about one-to-one casework, from a British and academic perspective. In my second year I worked with one case – a seven-year-old Afrikaner boy who'd been sexually abused by his mother's boyfriend – at a white primary school. My background was so different to this. The children's problems didn't relate to poverty. I once argued with my supervisor who asked us to get the children to play with Smarties. How can you play with food?

'It got more interesting when we started a new course on community work. I spent my third year at a clinic in a farming community. After checking it was alright with the big farmer and his wife, I started having meetings with the farm workers to help them set up a child-minding programme in the clinic, manned by *gogos* [grandmothers] I'd trained. I set it up! Yo!' She chuckles with satisfaction at her own achievement. 'Ya, that was good! Once we had the project up, the farmers' wives would know where to bring surplus milk or cracked eggs for the children. It's still going, I tell you. And now there's a school there. Ai!' She squeals with delight.

After graduating, Bongi returned to her hometown to work with children at a grim, church-funded institution. There were about 80 abandoned children aged from a few weeks to 18. Bongi set about trying to find parents for them all.

In the late 1980s and early 1990s, AIDS was barely mentioned in South Africa, but the problem of abandoned and orphaned children was growing. Many families in KwaZulu-Natal had been left bereaved and destitute by the political violence, but the impact of the epidemic would soon eclipse anything that had gone before. By 2010, there will be an estimated 500,000 orphans in this province of nine million people.

When she'd done her best for the institutionalised kids, Bongi the Baby Broker turned her attention to finding families for about 50 children who'd been abandoned at a local hospital.

'I'd go to the local magistrates' offices and there'd be lots of parents coming to pick up their state foster care grants, and I'd run monthly meetings for them. While I was talking about fostering and childcare, I'd also talk about the coming AIDS crisis. I'd ask them how they'd respond if they saw a child about to be hit by a car and then I'd tell them about all the abandoned children at the hospital.

'Can you believe that I actually managed to find parents who wanted HIV-positive kids? At one time there were eight, and I placed them all. It was like they'd accepted, "This is *our* problem. These are *our* children."'

Many South African social workers assume that black people don't want to take in unrelated children. They cite cultural reasons for blacks' seeming reluctance to foster and adopt in the past. Bongi's success at recruiting black parents suggests that systemic obstacles were probably more of an issue than any collective abhorrence of the idea. Many black families simply didn't know that they could adopt children, and others were told that they were unsuitable.

'A few years back, even the infertile didn't know that they could take in unrelated children', says Bongi. 'What had the social workers been doing? I became very unpopular with them. Even black social workers were saying I was throwing children away in the bush because they thought rural people didn't qualify to take children. I'd argue, "There's shelter, stability, food fresh from the garden and love."'

Julie Todd, director of the Child and Family Welfare Society in Pietermaritzburg, which matches abandoned children with foster parents, has watched her agency adapt. 'We now have different criteria for different communities', she says. 'If a black couple wants to adopt we're not as strict on the age limit or size of their house, because we have many more black children who need homes.' South African social workers are slowly learning to worry less about whether a client is a housewife with a childproof cover on her swimming pool and more about counting a family's livestock as indicators of family wealth.

Where cultural barriers to adoption did exist, Bongi, a Zulu herself, could sometimes persuade people round.

'The *gogos* [grandmothers] would worry that the personality of the abandoned child's father and ancestors were unknown to them. I'd ask, "What happens to illegitimate babies in our community? Are they thrown away?"

"No, no," say the *gogos*. "We take in that one, because it's part of us."

I'd say, "Good", and ask them, "What attributes are given to ancestors? OK, it's partly about family linkages but it's also how they led their life. If my grandpa was a killer, OK, he's an ancestor, but he's not a good spirit so I'll pay him no attention. I'll pray to good role-model ancestors because I want good will to continue to my children and my children's children." And I say, "Come on, this is our way out. If you want to take in a child crying in a dustbin and give it food and love, do you really think this is going against your ancestors?"

"No, not at all," they reply. Then I persuade them to do the same ritual, like slaughtering a chicken, that they would do if they were welcoming an illegitimate child into the family and introducing it to the ancestors.'

Infertility, the main reason why people decide to adopt unrelated children, holds a tremendous stigma in Africa. An infertile couple came to Bongi wanting to adopt a baby. The wife wanted to pad herself up and pretend to be pregnant for nine months to avoid being gossiped about. Bongi went along with it. In the end it took eleven months to find the couple a newborn.

As well as infertile couples, Bongi also had *gogos* wanting to foster children, especially those who'd been raising their grandchildren until their daughters suddenly whisked them away having decided they wanted their children to know their mother. The *gogos* miss the children.

Every couple of months, Bongi visits Mrs Zikalala, a *gogo* who decided to foster an HIV-positive child. Lindiwe is now three and lives with her elderly foster mother in Caluza, near the Edendale Valley. Mrs Zikalala took her into her home when her own two children were grown up. She points at Lindiwe and cackles, 'My third. Mandela's child', because Lindiwe was born, post-apartheid, during Nelson Mandela's presidency (1994–99).

Lindiwe was a sickly three-month-old baby when she arrived, but she has thrived. The old lady believes her herbs have cured the child and now sells them to other HIV sufferers. She finds some of the herbs locally, buys others from Zulu pharmacists, boils them up into a muddy-coloured solution and bottles it. The child gets four spoonfuls a day, plus a lot of love.

Mrs Zikalala's is one of the many poor homes that Bongi has placed children into despite colleagues' disapproval. It's a ramshackle place but a loving home. One of Mrs Zikalala's granddaughters is staying for a visit. The little girl strokes Lindiwe's sleeping head. She's fast asleep on a sofa and doesn't stir while Bongi visits. 'It's a very special thing to have a heart to take a child in', Bongi tells Mrs Zikalala as she leaves.

During the fighting in the Edendale Valley, many children were abandoned or orphaned. Some would be found and brought to

Edendale Hospital. Others would be admitted with ailments and then their families wouldn't return to pick them up when they were better. The nurses, already overburdened, often ignored them, so they'd lie four or five to a cot, unstimulated for hours.

Thandanani (meaning 'Love one another') was born in 1989 when a handful of volunteers started regularly coming to play with these children. Non-governmental organisations (NGOS) often emerge when caring individuals spot a social problem and get together to do something about it.

Within two years Thandanani had enough donations from overseas to hire three childcare workers to be permanently at the hospital. In 1994, all the nurses went on strike, basically abandoning the 80 children who'd already been abandoned on their wards. A concerted effort was made to find homes for the children. Bongi helped place many of them. The current director of Thandanani, Linda Aadnesgaard, adopted one.

Thandanani now has two programmes: a hospital programme dealing with abandoned babies and a community programme which sets up volunteer committees to keep an eye on needy children in townships and semi-rural areas. Bongi works on both.

The hospital programme is still needed to improve the quality of children's lives while they're hospitalised and to prevent the abandoned ones being neglected. At the moment, there are six children languishing at Edendale Hospital who shouldn't be there. Foster homes should have been found for them. Bongi shouts for their rights.

The hospital programme ticks along but Thandanani's main focus has switched to tackling AIDS orphans' problems out in the field. If Bongi personifies the shift in the focus of social work in South Africa, Thandanani represents the same shift within an organisation. It is an NGO that has observed the growing AIDS epidemic and tried to pre-empt some of the damage by setting up committees in communities that will, hopefully, be able to scoop up and assist the most needy orphans. NGOs, at their most dynamic, can change course much faster than governments.

In 1995 Dr Neil McKerrow, a paediatrician who saw the AIDS orphan crisis coming long before most of his compatriots, researched how people would respond to the problem in the Midlands area of KwaZulu-Natal. He found that 74 per cent of households would care for an AIDS orphan if it was a close relative, but only 42 per cent would take in an unrelated AIDS orphan. However, most felt that children should somehow be kept in their community of origin. This research informed Thandanani's change in direction. They decided to borrow the idea of building community childcare committees from Uganda, where the AIDS epidemic was a decade more advanced.

After consulting lots of people, they employed five fieldworkers and a co-ordinator to try to set up committees in nine areas to identify vulnerable children, help find surrogate families for orphans, report child abuse cases, persuade headteachers to take back children who had dropped out because they couldn't afford school fees and initiate projects like communal gardens, poultry farms and sewing groups to feed and clothe the poorest children.

The first problem was deciding what constituted a needy child. There were so many. Plus, AIDS was still taboo. Should they even be attempting to separate AIDS orphans from other vulnerable children? When asked to produce lists of names of orphans, committees would come back with other categories of needy children, invariably selected for their extreme poverty. There was a tension between letting communities decide their own criteria and subtly directing volunteers towards acknowledging the problems of AIDS orphans.

NGO workers can't just march into a community with their facts and figures and progressive ideas. There are ways to gain acceptance. Linda Aadnesgaard, who became Thandanani's first director in 1997, is refreshingly forthright. 'First of all,' she explains, 'what we have to do, which is a great big pain, is get the approval of the local elected councillor. They're supposed to be community leaders but they're notoriously inefficient.'

The councillors were more concerned with obtaining water, electricity and housing. Children didn't rate a mention in their list of concerns. Even when asked what specific problems children were encountering, communities talked about education, malnutrition and neglect, and not the fact that many were becoming orphans.

Linda continues,

'Once we've got past the councillors, we've gone into churches and women's groups to recruit volunteers to set up community childcare committees. Sometimes a broad community forum has elected them. Other times they've simply volunteered. But in both cases, we've found that people come along with the expectation of getting a job. We realise people are unemployed and poor, but there's no way we can pay them, not even a nominal amount because it creates a very difficult situation for us in terms of labour relations.'

South African employers don't take the decision to hire lightly, because it's virtually impossible to fire people. NGO funding is precarious, and if they had to lay staff off they would have to compensate them generously. Few NGOs can afford lots of staff anyway. Like most volunteer-dependent organisations, Thandanani struggles to retain and motivate them to work for nothing. People in the Edendale Valley are very poor.

Projects of this type are always a slow and tricky process. Families, already struggling to eat, are being asked to take on more, unrelated children. The act of setting up committees to identify vulnerable children sometimes raises unrealistic expectations. Even if the project's aims are carefully explained, many participants still assume that they are about to receive handouts. When they don't, they're disappointed and some committees fold. Volunteers find jobs, move away, lose interest and bicker. Three years on, six committees out of nine are still active.

Thandanani has experienced many setbacks.

'The first two years were a complete nightmare', admits Linda. 'There have been incredible learnings, but also within those learnings, a lot of negatives because you realise there are no quick and easy solutions. Government's spending money in all the wrong places. Basically it's got to go to where people are being given the burden of care; communities who are unemployed, impoverished, old and largely female.'

Part of Thandanani's difficulty in getting into the communities in the first place was because people had so many competing priorities. When democracy came to South Africa in 1994, people expected the new government to solve all their problems. They wanted cars, clinics, homes, schools, water, electricity and freedom. When these did not all materialise, they were disappointed. Nobody was even vaguely aware of what was coming next.

'And now,' sighs Linda, 'on top of everything else, we're going to have 50,000 AIDS orphans in this valley and the care for them is going to fall squarely on the shoulders of the poorest of the poor.

'We're only six years out of liberation. The new politicians promised a better life for all. Unions have also increased expectations and the entitlement culture. But the tax base is small. There simply aren't the resources. Unemployment, poverty and crime are up. Other countries have been independent for 20 years. South Africa is in a very different place.'

The new government felt pressurised to deliver quick, tangible results. In 1996, the Department of Health spent over R14 million (£1.4 million), a big chunk of the annual AIDS budget, on *Sarafina II*, a lavish musical to raise awareness of AIDS. Scandal broke when it became apparent that tendering procedures hadn't been followed. A high ticket price kept poor audiences out. It was an embarrassing, expensive flop.

Then in 1997, the government backed Virodene, a home-grown 'miracle' cure for AIDS, which turned out to be a harmful industrial solvent. When the Medicines Control Council refused to license clinical trials, the government purged the council.

In 1998, the government refused to provide AZT, an anti-retroviral drug, to HIV-positive pregnant women, even though it had been shown to reduce the risk of mother-to-child transmission by half. At first, the politicians complained that AZT cost too much. Then they claimed they were worried about the drug's toxicity although it had been approved in most Western countries. AIDS activists believe it would be cheaper than treating infected children later. Two years later, research in Uganda and South Africa on another drug for the same purpose, Nevirapine, showed that it was 50 per cent more effective than AZT, easier to administer and cheaper at R30 (£3) per mother and child. The government's continued reluctance to provide either of these drugs made activists furious.

One explanation is that the South African government was involved in a stand-off with the multinational drug companies, trying to win the right to bypass patent laws and buy cheap generic drugs. Perhaps they felt that agreeing to pay AZT's manufacturer, Glaxo Wellcome, even a heavily discounted price, would compromise South Africa's position as champion of the right of poor countries to ignore intellectual property laws protecting Western drug firms. Another possible obstacle to the provision of anti-retroviral drugs is South African president Thabo Mbeki's apparent doubts that the HIV virus causes AIDS.

The relationship between government and journalists, scientists and NGO workers has turned increasingly sour. Unlike in Uganda, few South African NGO workers say that they feel well-supported by government.

'There was a mass exodus of [black] people from NGOs into government after 1994,' says Linda, 'and the next most senior people were white. When we have to go and challenge government, we're all white. It's enormously problematic because we're so obsessed with race in South Africa. If we criticise them, we're told that we're anti-government and understand nothing ...'

Even as the HIV prevalence amongst pregnant women shot up from less than 1 per cent in 1990 to 23 per cent in 1998, government funding for AIDS NGOs was halved to R12 million (£1.2 million) that year. Some AIDS activists saw this as punishment for criticising the government over *Sarafina II*, Virodene and AZT.

During apartheid, foreign donors gave money directly to NGOs. After 1994, the new government encouraged donors to give them the money, promising to co-ordinate the NGOs. But much of the money doesn't get through. NGOs struggle to make ends meet.

The Department of Welfare spent about R16 billion (£1.6 billion) on social security grants in 1998, the bulk on old-age pensions. Even after deciding that they wanted to shift from providing handouts to services that encourage self-sufficiency, they realised that they couldn't stop paying pensions and foster care grants. They're too important a safety net. However, this leaves very little money for innovative development projects. The 600 or so NGOs that do AIDS-related work, do so on a shoestring.

The Department of Welfare is often ineffectual. It failed to spend more than a third of its national budget between 1996 and 1999 because of poor management. During 1998/99, it spent less than 1 per cent of its poverty relief funds.

The government has promised to investigate welfare benefits for families affected by HIV/AIDS and the possibility of subsidising adoption of AIDS orphans, but has set aside no budget for this.

Thandanani has received no funding from the government, although it fits nicely within the Welfare Department's professed priorities. In 1999/2000 Thandanani's total budget was R950,000 (£95,000), much of which came from foreign churches.

'Our committees expect there to be money', says Linda. 'They expect us to pay for their transport, catering and training courses – which we do. It's what we fundraise for, but there's an assumption about it and very little community spirit. There's clearly a need out there for someone to do something but nobody's sure who that somebody is. It's been a painful realisation that government's going to supply very little and people are going to have to do things for themselves. For me, this project's always been a challenge because the people we're pressurising the most are those who have the least.'

In the project's early days, when the newly formed committees had identified the most needy children in their area as requested, another problem arose. In South Africa, if you put your name down on a list, it's because there's something coming your way, like a housing benefit or a grant. Lists create expectations.

Quickly, before the project fell flat, Linda invented a series of 'campaigns' to help poor guardians deal with practical, usually material, problems like applying for child support grants (a new state benefit worth £10 a month for children under seven) and birth certificates for children (which are needed in order to get a grant). They helped grandmothers who'd had their pensions cut off and lobbied to get children back into school who'd dropped out.

Thandanani-style projects require clever management of volunteers, because otherwise donor funds might never reach the children they are supposed to benefit. A social worker at a well-established orphanage for HIV-positive children worries that money going 'into the community' achieves little because it becomes so diluted. 'We could scrap all that we're doing here [at the children's home] and the grant could go to the community, but there are such huge problems out there that it wouldn't really make an impact.'

The money Thandanani raises helps orphans by indirect methods such as paying for committee members to go on basic nursing, counselling or childcare courses. This keeps them motivated and gives them status in their communities.

On one occasion, Bongi drops in to say hello to 45 volunteers who are doing a first aid course. She speaks unselfconsciously in front of the crowd and makes them laugh as they dig into a lunch of rice and chicken. It's an in-depth course. Each person has been given a heavy textbook in English, although they speak Zulu and literacy levels vary. The volunteers want this training and some have recently attended a rape crisis course because they found that, as committee members, people come to them with all sorts of personal problems.

Bongi manages four fieldworkers whose job is to nurture the community committees. She has a weekly progress meeting with each. A session with Gugu Ndlela, one of the fieldworkers, is brief; just enough time to tell Gugu off for not producing regular written reports. Some of the staff find writing difficult. Bongi spends a lot of her day gently trying to exert some quality control over her staffs' work through good-natured nagging.

> 'Bongi is a Zulu so that's an advantage,' says Linda, 'but there's jealousy of her position and salary'.
>
> Linda lowers her voice so that her secretary won't hear her saying, 'All our staff are people from the community so the learning curve has been massive as their English isn't very good. We've been training them at the same time as trying to help the communities. This is reality. We're not going to have a whole lot of university graduates who'll dash out there with their little notebooks and set up community childcare committees. It's got to be done by ordinary people, but we didn't realise how difficult it would be.'

Thandanani's goal is to set up community childcare committees and then leave them to run themselves. But knowing when to let go is difficult. In fact, it's not clear whether poor communities will be able to look after all their needy children without external skills and money anytime soon.

Volunteers' motives are often complex. There's usually an element of altruism, but also the desire to get a job (or at least free training that might later get one a job) and the need for status in the community. All over the world, volunteers resent paid staff in charities.

When Thandanani secured funding to pay for school fees for 100 children, the board decided that committees should identify which ten children in their area were most in need. Linda thought this would increase volunteers' expectations. The board overruled her. A fraught general meeting followed during which volunteers accused Thandanani of being corrupt and sitting on money.

'Eventually they heard us saying, "These are *your* communities. These are *your* committees"' remembers Linda. 'They heard it, but with great pain because many of them have nothing.'

'Community mobilisation is incredibly important but we have to remember that our communities have been shattered by violence and poverty. I'm involved with a group who advise the Government's Inter-ministerial Committee about what they should do about AIDS orphans and they have the idea that communities are going to say, "Yes, of course we'll do it" to everything that's asked of them.'

Thandanani staff are more realistic. They used to go into a community and ask people to work. Now, they wait to be invited.

On a grey, rainy day, Bongi attends the first meeting of a new committee with fieldworker, Sipho Dlamini. Groups of bedraggled children coming out of school stand by the side of the road. 'You can identify the needy ones just by looking', comments Bongi. Some have uniforms, some have rags and others are almost naked. It's a desperately poor area. Most people are unemployed. Wattle and mud houses stick haphazardly half way up the sides of the valley. Minibus taxis, which recklessly race over the potholed muddy roads, provide the only means of transport.

Five ladies are waiting for Bongi and Sipho in the long grass outside a derelict building, a few parts of which have been reclaimed as offices. When local people want to get together, they clear out a room. Chairs are found and wiped clean.

Sipho tells the group straight out, 'I'm not Santa Claus arriving with lots of gifts.' The volunteers introduce themselves. Three are young mothers. Two are *gogos*. They're all dressed up for the occasion but they look shy and passive. Progress will be slow. Bongi leaves Sipho to get on with committee business or at least the business of deciding a name for their committee. Bongi quite often drops in on committee meetings, 'Because sometimes they don't happen.'

'The problem with development work,' says Bongi, 'is that you can't see it. We sow the seed, but I may be dead by the time our communities have developed their own infrastructures.'

Some people doubt that the AIDS orphan crisis will be contained by Thandanani-style projects alone. When an orphan is knocking at the door, starving, he can't be made to wait while communities slowly organise themselves into childcare committees.

In their first three years, it has proved impossible to establish enough committees to cope with the imminent crowd of AIDS orphans. But Linda believes their methods will catch on, as more people die and their neighbours wake up to the crisis. Meanwhile, staff at Thandanani need patience not to be discouraged by the poverty and suspicion they encounter daily. NGO workers have to support communities' own ways of coping, without wading in and undermining their efforts. There's no quick and easy route to self-reliance.

Despite all the set-backs, Linda and Bongi still believe that their community model could be scaled up. Certainly it has the potential to reach more children than are formally fostered, adopted or institutionalised. In 2000, the Department of Welfare is paying Linda to visit six other provinces to talk to people about setting up similar projects. Thandanani doesn't want the responsibility for the success or failure of the new sites. They're just offering to share what they have learnt.

A degree in social work didn't prepare Bongi for the task of organising volunteers into committees, but she relishes the challenge.

'I never dreamt that my childminding project would grow into a primary school in the farming community where I spent my third year of college. But the community took it, got funding and made it happen. This is what I want to see here: day-care centres for children, run by volunteer committees, like central points in every community. If anyone wants to donate something, run an HIV prevention campaign or a soup kitchen, they'd know where to go to reach the children. It would be for all children, but with special attention given to the needy ones. This is my vision. It's still in my head, but, for me, it's the future.'

5
Hope in the hills

'Cluster Fostering' in Rural KwaZulu-Natal, South Africa

'I saw a group of children. They looked strangely quiet. I said, "Who are these children?" And Tim, my guide, said, "Oh these are the AIDS orphans." They looked starving. They couldn't reach the fruit, which grows along every road in Uganda. I said, "This is dreadful", and went to get our lunch for them from the car.

'I went into one of the huts and there was a child dying on the floor, tummy out to here. I was totally unprepared for this. Tim was saying, "But this is happening all over Uganda at the moment." It was 1992.

'I said, "God, no, this should never happen." On a planet that spends billions on arms and space programmes, no child should ever die alone. And suddenly I knew what my life was going to be: working to save the children.

'At the time, I couldn't let go and be hysterical because I was with people who'd come to terms with this. I went back to Kampala and phoned Patrick, my husband. Then I could cry. I said we had to go to Uganda and work for the children. He said I should come home to South Africa and we'd discuss it.'

God's Golden Acre, a 'cluster' foster home for orphaned and abandoned children, set amongst rolling hills on Cato Ridge in South Africa's KwaZulu-Natal province, is the result of this revelatory moment in Heather Reynolds' life. She tells the story with enthusiasm.

'When Patrick and I were in our twenties, I looked in the newspaper and there was an old house for rent out in the bush. It was the most beautiful, run-down place about two kilometres from the road. I said, "Let's forget the ugliness of the world." We quit our office jobs and concentrated on our art. Patrick sculpts. I paint. We had hard times ahead and I was an atheist at that time, but it was quite an idyllic life.'

Heather's life has been full of significant moments.

'Then came a moment when my whole life turned upside down. My brakes failed at a stop sign and I went straight into a car, with my baby in the back. It spun me and I went off the road. Amazingly, we were both fine and as I walked up the road, two men came down. I was waiting for the abuse. Instead a gentle voice said, "Are you OK?" And I said, "Fine, are you?" And they said, "Fine." And the driver said, "Let's just say a prayer." And it blew my mind. I'd left a charismatic church in my teens that had left me scarred. But this was true Christianity, to say, "Never mind my brand new imported Jaguar sports car", which I'd written off. I thought maybe there is a God. And I wondered if I could ever be like that.'

The opportunity to do good works came unexpectedly.

'Not long after that, the first little girl came to us. She was 14 and very pregnant. She came to our farm asking for work. She said, "I have nobody. I had a granny but now she's dead." I said to Patrick, "We can't have her in the house, but what are we going to do with her?" and he said, "Why not?"'

It was the early 1980s and Heather knew how difficult it would be to take a black person into her home. In apartheid South Africa, many whites wouldn't eat off the same plates or use the same bathrooms as their black compatriots. Heather was living in Umvoti, a conservative German area of what was then called Natal province.

'I knew our community. If you were seen with a black person after dark you were thrown in jail ... But we took her in. There was no other choice. And her baby was born on Christmas Day. My family has never visited since that day 18 years ago. They still love me but, no way, they wouldn't come into my house.'

Heather and Patrick fell upon bad times. She had to have several operations and they had no medical insurance. Then they lost all their money in a panel-beating business. They were broke.

'We hit rock bottom. And my mind turned to God. Strange things were happening. Another pregnant teenager came to us asking for work. And then another. Eventually I had eight of them, aged 14 or 15. I'd look after the babies while they went back to school. The crèche just grew although we had no money.'

Heather got caught up in the civil strife that raged in the KwaZulu and Natal region during the 1980s and 1990s because she'd got to know the relatives of the teenagers she'd taken in. They lived in a valley that was badly affected.

'One cold, wet night, 38 refugees turned up on my veranda; people who'd been burnt out of their homes. Some of them were from the IFP [Inkatha Freedom Party]. Others were from the other side [the African National Congress]. They'd come to us because their daughters knew me. We put them up in a barn. I got bedding and potatoes from friends in town. Not from the local community. My landlord would not have been happy if he'd known what we were doing. They couldn't go back because the violence continued.'

With almost 50 people to feed, Heather needed money. She heard about a company who needed someone to sell an asphalt plant in Uganda. No one had applied for the job, despite the offer of a hefty R60,000 (about £6,000) commission. It was the time of the genocide in neighbouring Rwanda; people were scared. But not Heather. Without friends, contacts or a plan of action, she set off.

'I was late for the plane and had to run. There was one seat left next to a lady called Avril. I was telling her about my task and she said, "My husband works for the Ugandan government. He's coming to fetch us and he'll arrange for you to meet the minister of transport." They invited me to stay and arranged everything. I then had several days to kill before my appointment, so my hosts lent me their bodyguard, Tim and their four-by-four, so I could do some sightseeing.

'One day we'd gone about 250 kilometres, somewhere in the east near Mbale, and I said I needed some water. No one had checked that the kitchen staff had put it in the boot. Tim said there was a natural spring nearby, which would be safe to drink from. We walked through the forest and that's where I met the AIDS orphans ...'

This chance encounter changed everything.

'On the way home, in a Nairobi hotel room, I asked God for help. I was an artist and knew I'd always be poor, but now I needed money to start an orphanage in Uganda. I decided to write a letter to the press to let them know what I'd seen. I said, "God, I'm not a writer. You've got to help me." Instead of giving me a letter, God gave me lyrics. Suddenly I was writing a song. I'd never written one before. It was a miracle.'

Years later, at God's Golden Acre, Heather calls in some of the children to sing it with her:

> Give a child a home
> Give a child a home
> Don't let them die all alone
> On God's Golden Acre
> They'll get to know their Maker
> Give a child a home.

She returned to South Africa, and was busy persuading Patrick to go to Uganda when a television programme about AIDS came on. A paediatrician called Neil McKerrow was being interviewed about the statistics for AIDS orphans in South Africa. Heather tuned in.

'Patrick and I hadn't been reading newspapers. We didn't want to see the violence. Obviously we'd heard of AIDS but we hadn't got hold of it. And here, suddenly, we were hearing what was going to be happening in South Africa over the next decade. It blew my mind. I thought, "I must speak to this man." When the credits came up, it said, "Phone Dr McKerrow at Edendale Hospital." He was down the road!'

Dr McKerrow suggested that instead of an orphanage in Uganda, she start a 'cluster foster care scheme' where she was. It would reach more children.

In the early days, God's Golden Acre was little more than one woman looking after 35 needy children in a small, overcrowded house with an outside toilet. Sometimes, there would be a two-hour queue for the bathroom. They were desperately hard up, especially when their cars were stolen.

South Africa is one of the most unequal societies on earth. Heather grows incensed when she talks about the disparity of wealth in her area. In the early days of God's Golden Acre, she had terrible difficulties finding enough money to feed children and, at one time, no car to transport a dying baby to hospital, despite living in an affluent community.

'The German farmers in Wartburg own so much and the rural communities have nothing. The farmers never really go down into the valleys. They just drive through in their Mercedes.

'People would ask me why I'm wasting people's time and money on these kids. One man told me to, "Put the whole damn lot of them down a mine shaft and, do me a favour, seal it to make sure those things don't come out."

'One time I was in the taxi rank with the kids singing. I'd made a placard saying, "God's Golden Acre cares about our orphans. Jesus taught us to love. Why are you not loving?" Our Pastor came and joined me. We marched to the church hall where he'd organised a meeting.

'And I blew my top in front of the congregation. I said, "Why do I have to beg you for a lift to take my dying child to hospital?" I told them, "I don't want to be part of this community. I've had it." And a voice at the back said, "I think I can take care of your transport problem." He comes up to me and puts the keys for a Toyota truck in my hand.'

A little while later, Heather found the perfect site to build her 'cluster foster care scheme'. Friends and family gave her the money to put a deposit down on the place she'd call Khayelihle (Beautiful Home). When she showed her management committee the ramshackle farm on the top of a hill, they thought she was mad. 'It was so run-down when we arrived,' she says, 'but we've had diggers clearing the place and there's now running water and electricity'.

Building work will continue for months, maybe years. But an amazing amount has already been accomplished. Here, foundations are being laid. There, a pig shed is being turned into accommodation for eight kids. A temporary schoolhouse has been made more permanent. There are plans for a dining room. Heather can picture how it will be. She can see a whole community covering the hill, down into the valley and up over the next hill. There will be houses for orphans, disabled and elderly people. When grandmothers can no longer cope, they may come with their orphaned grandchildren and be supported, maybe taking on a few extra children too. How will they all subsist? Heather plans an art gallery, a nursery, bead work, ethnic dancing and all manner of other enterprises.

God's Golden Acre is far removed from anyone's idea of a traditional orphanage. The setting is spectacular. Twenty-two children live in clusters with six foster mothers. Heather gets calls from people in hospitals or down in the valley when an abandoned baby's been found. She frequently finds the children in horrific circumstances. Some have been sexually abused or seen their parents die. Some arrive covered with pus-filled sores. Others are like feral cats, biting and spitting.

Heather and Patrick sleep in the main farmhouse. Opposite the front door are outhouses where foster mums sleep, each in a crowded room with their charges. It's a homely, chaotic set-up. People wander in and out of the farmhouse. One of seven cats lies curled up in the middle of a cluttered table. There are boxes everywhere. A baby called Mandla lies in one of them, barely breathing. It was his first birthday yesterday. There's a net over him to keep out the flies and traces of vomit on a rag by his mouth. He looks sick and miserable. He's been close to death in recent days.

Surrounded by children in the main farmhouse, Heather points out, 'That's little Jabulile, who was shot by her father. He put her face down and shot her through her spine. We saved her leg. A surgeon from Johannesburg came out and operated on our kitchen table.' Jabulile takes off her shoe to show Heather a raw, wet wound on her foot. She's clearly had an ulcer there for a while, but because she has no feeling in it, the infection's reached the bone. 'No more swimming, Jabulile. Get those wet shoes off, Jabulile', she chides.

A small boy climbs onto her lap. 'It's such a privilege to hold this little fella, Hlengiwe. He was found alone in a room. He was seven months and if you put your finger anywhere near him, he'd bite you. They thought he was retarded, but he's three now and he's fine, just small; smaller than a two-year-old.'

The children call her *Gogo* (Granny). In the evening, after their baths, she announces, 'It's family time', and they all come into the main farmhouse and try to sit on her. Heather doesn't seem to need privacy, except perhaps when mourning.

'I've lost five children in the last six years. It doesn't get easier, but it doesn't get cumulatively worse either. Somehow you put the grief away … I remember each child clearly.

'Sarah was a tiny doll. She was beautiful. I grieved for the fact that she was never able to run or walk or play.

'Jolly was five and a half. I was able to talk to her about her pain and tell her about a place where there was no pain.' Heather's voice falls to a whisper. 'I can't talk any more …'

She cries for the children she has cared for who have died.

About seven of the 22 kids are HIV-positive. They're all doing OK, except Mandla in his little box.

All of the children have been orphaned or abandoned, so God's Golden Acre has become their home. They're unlikely to be fostered or adopted by ordinary families, because they are HIV-positive, disabled or traumatised. As they grow older however, other options sometimes arise. Heather has recently returned a group of five siblings to their family home. There are no adults in the picture, but with support from God's Golden Acre, they're now going it alone.

'From the beginning, we'd left Peter, who's 16, in the family home, to hold on to it', explains Heather. 'There are about six huts in their *kraal* [homestead] and that's their heritage. We used to send the other four younger children home every holiday so they'd be together as a family.

'And then Rachel went home to join Peter. That was hard. She's 13 now. They're both still in school. She was about nine when we first took her and it took four years to launch her back into her family. I encouraged her because I thought Peter needed it. He'd been on his own, except for his older brother, Musa. But Musa had gone off to Durban and we couldn't find him for a while. Now we've even got him to come home. I don't see that much of them any more because I'm so busy here. I'm just sending them food and clothes now.

'Letting the little ones go back was the hardest thing. But like with Rachel, I had to let them go. They were becoming too close to us and losing their relationship with their family. The youngest, Nomsa, is four now and can go into pre-primary. Khehla is five and Phumuzile is eight. As they're all in school, no one is left alone during the day to be abused. Musa's back and bringing in a bit of income as he gets *tok* [temporary jobs] at the mill. But I think it will fall on Rachel, as the oldest girl, to hold it together, although Peter's a pretty responsible boy. They're an incredible little family.'

Heather is keen to engineer new families out of the remnants of those torn apart by AIDS. She wants to put more women, and especially grandmothers, who themselves need food and shelter, to work caring for orphans.

'As we find more abandoned or orphaned children, we'll bring them here and get them healthy again. Then if we find a granny who's willing, maybe we'll be able to place them with that granny. We'll then take food, nappies and clothing twice a month and check everything's OK. If a granny has, say, two or three orphans and really can't cope, she could come and live here and then we'd let her take another three children to make up a cluster.'

Heather is just beginning to experiment with combining families. 'We've got two *gogos* [grandmothers] who might become foster mums, but what we've done with one is to put her back into a hut in the valley where there's another *gogo* living alone with a child. The two *gogos* didn't know each other before, but they seem to be getting on.'

One sunny afternoon, Heather and Patrick are wandering around the farm outbuildings, stumbling over roots and bits of concrete. Five dogs, all shapes and sizes, play exuberantly in the long grass. Heather and Patrick are discussing the future of each building because the provincial housing department has recently donated a million rand (about £100,000) to help Heather realise her dream of creating a new community of 72 people who'll live in six brand new three-bedroom homes. The windfall has thrown all plans up in the air.

'The principle of cluster foster care will apply at the new site too', says Heather, proudly. 'They'll be a group of foster mums living in close proximity, depending on each other. They'll have semi-detached homes with connecting doors so if one foster mum is ill or needs time off, there'll be another next door who'll be able to look after the children. And they won't be far from us. There'll also be a separate hospice building so if any of the children get very sick, they can go there, but it won't be far removed from their siblings.'

Some people question the wisdom of the provincial housing department's decision. The government doesn't normally fund the building of orphanages.

Heather is planning a veranda at Khayelihle with a sweeping view of the surrounding hills. She also wants a nice room for entertaining foreign donors. They discuss where Patrick will have his studio and where they'll live. Heather's being bossy. Patrick's grumpy. He's not happy with the building that she has in mind for his studio. She half-jokingly reminds him that if she's bringing in a million rand at a time now, his sculptures are no longer the primary breadwinner.

Another of Heather's money-making schemes is to invite groups of schoolchildren to come out to the Khayelihle 'resort'. They play on the water slide, roast sausages on the *braai* (barbecue) and go on pony rides and nature trails. In the future Heather expects tourists to come. She encourages the foster mothers to learn arts and crafts skills, so that they will be able to sell curios to tourists.

An engineer called Craig wandered in one day. When Heather showed him where she was planning a vegetable garden, he pointed out that it wouldn't work under eucalyptus trees. He's now coming back to do it for them, and will do the same at the new site. He'll train the teenagers in agricultural skills. Heather wants God's Golden Acre to feed itself. There are also three volunteer teachers and Heather plans to bring in older girls from the valley and train them to be schoolteachers too.

God's Golden Acre now has four 'satellites'. They're autonomous projects (or simply compassionate individuals fostering a number of needy children in their own homes) but Heather gives them moral, and occasionally financial, support.

Heather is used to encountering scepticism when she lays out her grand vision, so she hesitates to fix a timetable. She becomes defensive if she feels someone is not with her. 'It's easier to explain to people who believe, because they don't think I'm crazy', she explains. She asks everyone if they are Christian, and it worries her if they're not. Her evangelism puts some people off.

In the mid-1990s, Mark Loudon ran Children in Distress (CINDI), an umbrella organisation for non-governmental organisations (NGOs) concerned about vulnerable children in KwaZulu-Natal. God's Golden Acre is an active member. A few years on, Mark remembers how Heather runs her organisation. 'Heather kept changing her mission. One time it might be, "We need funding for an airline ticket to go to America to sell my husband's sculpture to get money to run our children's home." The next time, it might be something completely different. It became hair-raising.'

Mr Loudon doesn't believe that God's Golden Acre is something that could be scaled up to meet the magnitude of the coming AIDS orphan crisis in South Africa.

'Heather's doing a great job but let's not fool ourselves that it's replicable. It's not. It's entirely run on her spirit, guts and energy. And it's great. But it's important that people don't attach a greater significance to it, believe it's how we should run our response to the orphan crisis. A project like that can fail just as easily as it can succeed. There's no idea so good that it can survive bad management. And in her case, she's got some fairly shocking ideas. But they work. Because she's behind them.'

Others disagree. They believe that the housing of AIDS orphans in 'clusters' is replicable and the best way to use and support whatever human resources – grandmothers, widows, HIV-positive mothers – are left looking after the growing numbers of needy children. Some use the term 'kibbutz' to describe such idealistic, collective efforts but Heather says, 'No, I'm not a kibbutz. Not at all. Not at all. We're a cluster foster community centre.'

People who know Heather praise her energy but worry that she isn't very focused. Big one-off donations apart, her fundraising efforts are a little erratic. She believes God will provide. Meanwhile, she counts out Herbalife products (homeopathic pills sold, pyramid-fashion, out of people's homes) into a box whilst talking to someone on the phone who will sell them on for her. She had bought R4,000 (£400) worth to try to make a quick profit but hadn't found the time to sell them. She also sells artwork and bonsai trees. Despite having acquired beautiful space at Khayelihle, the whole operation still feels hand to mouth.

'There are times when perhaps I'm a bit emotional and have a bit of a set-to with my committee', says Heather. 'I'll say I'm here to look after the children and they'll be trying to encourage me to take only children who have papers and come with a state grant. But in the valley, children don't have birth certificates. And if they're at death's door, there's no way I'm going to worry about … by tomorrow that child might be dead. So then I just have to forcefully say that the paperwork and the money will have to come later. Right now, tonight, that child is in need and I'll take it and bring it home.'

Feeding everybody at God's Golden Acre is a major operation. The team of foster mums does the cooking, washing and cleaning.

'Our foster mums are people from the valley who I've been working with for many years', says Heather. 'Some of them are the girls I helped in the past when they were pregnant teenagers. We've grown up together. They know this is a mission station. They get some work and they're doing something for God. I don't have problems with them asking for money or overtime because they know I don't have a salary. We give them a small retainer of R500 [about £50] a month, free clothes, food and accommodation and two weeks' leave. If something happens at their family's home, we go and find out what's cooking. If a relative of theirs dies we help move the body.'

Thandi has been working for Heather for 14 years. She's a calm, obliging woman.

'I met Mrs Reynolds in 1989 when I was a young girl', she says. 'I heard about her through a woman who was working for her. She talked to Mrs Reynolds about me looking for a job. I worked in her garden with the plants and the bonsai. Then she told me about her idea for a home for the orphans. I wanted to be involved from the beginning. I became one of her foster mothers in 1998. I enjoy it. I'm on the committee now.'

Thandi went away to get trained in needlework, but came back. This is her home.

'When the children go to school, I clean inside the farmhouse and the nursery. We foster mothers help each other and do the washing together. But the best thing is looking after the children; caring for them and keeping them clean. At the moment, my six children are well. But I've had two die in the last year. It's hard but the foster mothers look after each other.'

There's a phone call for Thandi. Her 32-year-old cousin has died leaving four orphans. The youngest is two. Another cousin of hers died two months previously and Thandi's already paying the school fees of the two orphans left behind.

Thandi wanders out of the farmhouse, looking stunned.

God's Golden Acre will probably grow and get more organised, because it fires people's imagination. They hear about it; call Heather, donate things and volunteer their time. She's never advertised for volunteers, but they keep arriving. There's a gang of eight fresh-faced, young volunteers from Japan, Germany and England. They're giving a year of their life to Heather's cause. Plus it's a travelling experience for them.

A teenager called Nonhlanhla joins Heather on a veranda at the back of the farmhouse. She wears a tartan dress, tight curls and an unhappy expression. She's 13 and has been at God's Golden Acre since she was eleven. She's one of Thandi's six charges.

Her mother was hit by a minibus taxi and killed about 18 months ago. She didn't know her father. She has two younger brothers. One's eight, the other a severely disabled baby. Heather says,

'The youngest was fine but now he has cerebral palsy and HIV. He was fine till about seven months ago, just before we got him. I'm not sure what caused it, whether it was meningitis or what, but now he's blind and disabled. He was on his deathbed.

'When Nonhlanhla came, she was a wild street child. She was only eleven but everybody was terrified of her. All the other kids were from the valleys, you know, just little, orphaned kids, but she was a tough girl from a township, and she'd been raped. One time, she stabbed another child, Peter, through the chest, and nearly killed him. They were playing outside and he must have got too rough with her or something. At one point, I really thought we couldn't cope with her. I physically shook her and said, "Listen to me. You've got to change, Nonhlanhla, or I've got to let you go." But we stuck with it and she has become like my own daughter. She comes into my bedroom every morning to give me a big hug.'

Nonhlanhla considers questions for a long time. She sometimes needs a minute to sort out her thoughts. It's difficult to know whether this is due to difficulty with English, shyness or other emotions. Finally, she says, 'I live with Thandi. I am one of six here. I have two brothers and the others are little too. I am the oldest one. I help the little ones.'

When her mother died, her aunt took her to a social worker who brought her and her brothers to God's Golden Acre.

'It was OK, but overcrowded when we lived in Wartburg. It was small, but now everything is better. There's a pool and a slide.' Like so many orphans who've been at the receiving end of social services, she wants to be a social worker and work with children.

Her aunt doesn't visit. 'They live far away', she says wistfully. A few of the other children have relatives who come and most have somewhere else to go for Christmas. Nonhlanhla and her brothers don't. How does she feel about this? She sits in silence. Her head droops and suddenly big tears are rolling down her cheeks. Heather holds her.

Nonhlanhla is old enough to realise what she's been through and what she's lost. She carries a weight of responsibility for her brothers. She bends over the baby's pram, positioning a net to keep flies off. She's become a caring child. The unconditional love she has received here has allowed her to let down her guard a bit. She might benefit from professional counselling, but it is unlikely she will receive it. Nonhlanhla gets care here, but not therapy.

Heather murmurs that it is good for her to cry. Nothing makes up for the loss of her mother but she knows they all care about her at God's Golden Acre. The girl sits with her head down, her legs hanging loosely, toes pointing in; a picture of misery.

'It's a mess. It really is', says Heather. She could be talking about Nonhlanhla's life or the loss of five babies she's loved or the whole AIDS epidemic. God's Golden Acre is a beautiful, chaotic place, full of love and care but also some awfully traumatised children. The younger ones seem happy enough playing on climbing frames. But one or two lie pathetically, terminally sick and the older children like Nonhlanhla just look terribly sad. Everything pivots on Heather. On a day when fog shrouds the hills, her creation, God's Golden Acre, smells of urine, dirty laundry and wet dog. On a sunny day, when noisy, happy kids play football with volunteers, the place seems quite idyllic.

Sitting on the veranda, Heather suddenly remembers another piece of her story,

'You know, I never did get the commission from selling the asphalt plant in Uganda. I got the deal and then I waited for them to pay up. I even went up to Johannesburg to ask for it but they'd gone bust. I was very angry but by then my mind was on the orphans. I had other things to get on with. And you know, when we needed a new chairman, I told the committee that we needed to wait for God to give us the right man. After five months, our vice chair said he'd found us one. It turned out to be Alan McCarthy, the man who said a prayer after I'd written off his beautiful car.'

6
Institutionalised

An Orphanage in Cape Town, South Africa

Mandisi is a little doughnut of a child. He grins a lot and he knows he's being funny when he tells people he's six (he's actually four). He has a big appetite and a big tummy. He also has well-honed 'like-me' skills, which are useful because he is the latest addition at Beautiful Gate, a new orphanage for HIV-positive children in Crossroads, a township on the outskirts of Cape Town in South Africa.

His favourite adult is Ziyekele the cook, a big, warm woman with a smile that reveals a missing front tooth. 'You give me meat so you be my mama', he tells her.

Ziyekele talks to Mandisi in Xhosa. He tells her what little he knows about himself. He knows he was born in Khayelitsha, a nearby township. But he does not know where his mum is, or his dad. As he talks, he grows tense. He clutches a wooden puzzle to his forehead. This discussion is making him stressed and sad, so Ziyekele changes the subject. It is not surprising that he has picked her out. She's a maternal woman with five grandchildren of her own. She's also in charge of his food supply.

When Mandisi arrived, almost nothing was known about him. A social worker brought him and said she was not taking him away. He did not even have medical records. The staff still don't know whether he has tuberculosis or not. He coughs a lot at night. Despite coming from another children's home, he arrived at Beautiful Gate like a little parcel with no label attached.

Frances Herbert is the social worker at Beautiful Gate. She has found out a few more details about Mandisi.

'He's been with us for a month now. He came from a home run by the Child Welfare Society in Khayelitsha. They just closed it. He was there from a very early age because he was abandoned. He has got a mother but she's a vagrant. I don't know when anyone last saw her. He used to go to his wheelchair-bound father but he hasn't phoned or seen the child this year. I don't think Mandisi has any siblings. So that's where he's coming from.

'But he's settled in. I think he clicked from the moment he came. Although he sometimes cried to try and get something. He's the oldest child here and you can tell he's come from another home because he knows *everything*!'

Sian Hasewinkel of Cape Town's Child Welfare organisation, which is a fostering and adoption agency as well as running a children's home, explains why they had to close Mandisi's old home,

'Finance. Pure and simple. We're close to half a million rand [about £50,000] in deficit. If we'd continued to run it, we'd have folded in a couple of years.

'Children's homes definitely have their place but the problem is that once children go into them, it's very hard to get them out again. Social workers tend to think the child is placed, so they can now focus on the 60 others who aren't. They're also incredibly expensive. The state gives R800 [£80] a child per month to a children's home compared to R350 [£35] for foster care grants, so you can see why the government's not wildly keen.'

The South African government wants to keep AIDS orphans in their own communities rather than dumped in expensive institutions. So when Toby and Aukje Brouwer opened Beautiful Gate at the end of 1999, the state did not help them.

Cape Town is in the Western Cape, South Africa's southernmost province. It has the lowest prevalence of HIV/AIDS in the country. In 1999, 7 per cent of pregnant women attending antenatal clinics there were HIV-positive compared to 33 per cent in KwaZulu-Natal, the country's most stricken province.

Crossroads is half an hour from Cape Town's beaches, cafés and buzzing business district, but a world apart. The people here live in rows of makeshift shacks surrounded by steaming piles of rubbish. Skinny dogs scavenge. There are mountains in the distance, but Crossroads is on flat and dry land. Fast, hot winds pick up dust and litter and throw it along the main road and into people's eyes.

Beautiful Gate is set back from the main road. A security guard watches the unremarkable entrance. There are spacious gardens around a group of sturdy, red brick residential blocks. It's a little green oasis. The lives of the eight small children living here are, materially, better than those of the children who live the other side of the high fence. However, the young residents are sickly and cut off from family life.

Frances describes how it got off the ground.

'This is the second home set up by Toby and Aukje. The first one, which started in 1994, is for street children. This one is for HIV and AIDS babies. A year ago they found this beautiful spot. It was a children's home before, but the previous people found better premises so it was just standing empty. It was in such a state. Shattered. Broken windows. It took them nine months to make the place as it is now. They had to paint, replace the windows and bathrooms. They worked so hard to get everything ready, ordering all the medication, porridge and nappies. It was like preparing for a new baby coming home.

'Then in September 1999, the rest of us came on board. They advertised in the newspaper for a Christian social worker that knows about AIDS and speaks Xhosa. I phoned and said, "Listen, I have no knowledge of either of the two things that you request." And they said, "None of us knows anything about AIDS. We're all learning."

'We had 14 days of training covering home nursing, death and dying, team work and how to work with children. By 20 September, we had this beautiful place and trained staff ready, but no children. My job was to get them in.'

When orphanages open, like a vacuum, they soon fill up. Frances continues,

'The first child, Bulelwa, was placed with us on the 27 September. He spent nearly a month with us before the second request came. It was a little girl called Beauty who'd been abandoned. The two of them were here for three weeks before all the other children came. We now have eight children, from eleven months to four and a half years. I have a waiting list of children but we don't have the staff to take more at the moment.

'We're working on a two-year plan with our children. If, after that time, a child is well and there's a family member who's fit, the child will be placed back with them. If the mum is not well, there's usually an aunt. I'm not thinking of grandmothers because I think they're too old. These children will always be sick, so they need someone healthy to care for them. If there's no family, they will either stay on here or we can try and place them in foster care.'

Most of the children will die by the age of five. If they're still alive at seven, difficult decisions about their future will have to be made.

If no family has been found, they'll have outgrown Beautiful Gate and will have to be transferred to another orphanage for older children. This worries Frances. But it's a problem for the future. At the moment, she wants to believe that there's a home out there for every child.

> 'We are praying that there will be families in the local communities who will be prepared to foster HIV-positive children', she says. 'We would train and support them but it's difficult to know whether foster families will be able to cope.
>
> 'Our vision is that we will eventually care for 60 children, aged nought to six. I think it will take about a decade, because if I look at Nazareth House they have 43 children and I think they've been going for quite some time.'

Nazareth House is the other Cape Town institution exclusively for HIV-positive children. It was started, for a different purpose, in the 1880s. Over the years, it has been a vast Victorian orphanage, a home for the elderly, older children and then younger ones and, since 1998, a home for HIV-positive children. They admitted their first HIV-positive child seven years ago. This child is still with them. In fact, they now have three seven-year-olds who have recently started primary school.

Nazareth House has never managed to place an HIV-positive child with foster parents. Occasional enquiries have come to nothing.

The imposing convent is in the leafy suburb of Vredehoek under Table Mountain. It is run by six nuns in pristine white wimples. As well as 43 children under seven, they also care for 70 elderly people. The two groups do not mix. They are building space for an additional 20 children, without government support. Toby Brouwer went there for advice many times prior to launching Beautiful Gate. The two homes have a similar ambience.

In 1997, five of the children at Nazareth House died. In 1998, they lost another five and in 1999 they lost three. Jane Payne, the social worker there, explains why they do not separate the very sick children from the healthy.

> 'It's their home. It's not a medical facility. If they're really sick they go to hospital but the doctors send them back saying there's nothing more they can do. Then they stay here in one of the rooms. It means that everybody they know and care about, and

who cares about them, is there. We try and make sure there's somebody with them 24 hours. We don't feel it's necessary to have a special hospice section. Generally they seem to die during the night, so the children aren't seeing coffins brought in.

'The children don't ask many questions. Our policy is to answer anything as honestly as we can, but they don't ask. They'll say, "Where's Peter?" and you explain but that will be it. At four or five, they ask lots of "Why?" questions but not about AIDS. It's not avoided. It just doesn't come up.

'They may talk about their friends who have died. There's a picture of them and they'll say, "Peter died" but they're too young to have a real concept of what death's about. But they definitely miss their little friend. They all cry quite a bit but they'll have seen the little one get sicker and sicker. It happens slowly. It's become part of their lives.'

Staff at orphanages know that they're working against the tide. They acknowledge that they should be a last resort, but firmly believe that children's homes have an important role to play in the coming AIDS orphans crisis.

'If orphanages don't exist, what's going to happen to these children?' asks Jane. 'They're going to die. I know it's not right but I can see, like in the old days, huge big orphanages having to open up. Otherwise children will starve and there will be masses of street children.'

Frances at Beautiful Gate tries to keep in touch with outside social workers who work with the impoverished, AIDS-stricken families the other side of the fence. Some of the children have mothers and relatives living nearby so, in theory, could go home to see them. In practice only two children have ever been out for weekends with their families.

Frances would like to see an organisation formed that could help single HIV-positive mothers and their children stay together as long as possible.

'At the kind of set-up I envisage, they could be independent, work while they still can and their children could go to a crèche. This isn't what we're doing here but this would be my vision. We should be able to say to them, "Phone us if you can't cope." Because most of these children land up in hospital and that's where the mothers abandon them because they see there's medical care and somebody feeding their baby.'

The stigma around AIDS is still pervasive in South Africa. People have reason to be afraid of revealing their HIV status. People are often fired for being HIV-positive, although such discrimination is illegal. HIV can also lead to ostracism, or worse. In December 1998, a young AIDS activist, Gugu Dlamini, was stoned to death by her neighbours after she bravely revealed that she was HIV-positive on television. Her killers believed that she had brought their township into disrepute. They have still not been brought to justice.

Some of the mothers of children at Beautiful Gate are so afraid of their families finding out that they're HIV-positive that they refuse to visit their children. They don't want to be spotted leaving a children's home for HIV-positive children. Some of them are in denial. Frances is bemused,

'You know, I think that most of these mothers don't even know their child is HIV because they come and say, "What is this place for?" And you say, "This is for HIV children", and they say, "Is my child HIV?" I don't know how they don't know. Perhaps they just push it out of their mind. You know, I'm not sure they've even registered that they're HIV.

'Some of them get confused,' she continues, 'and think their child is coming to live here permanently. It's difficult because I speak English and Afrikaans and the mums speak Xhosa. The outside social workers must explain to them that after two years we have to make a recommendation to the court as to whether the child can go back home or why, for medical reasons or whatever, the child must stay with us.'

The kids are very sickly. They have a maximum of two or three weeks being well and then fall ill again. 'Most of them have chest problems, either tuberculosis or pneumonia', says Frances. 'Diarrhoea comes and goes. Fever comes and goes. At the moment, four are doing OK but the other four are struggling.'

At Nazareth House, where there are 43 sickly children, the staff fight a constant war against illness. Fungal infections cause painful, fluid-filled pustules all over children's bodies. If one child gets chicken pox, they all do. They recover, and then another bug assaults their immuno-compromised bodies.

Beautiful Gate's youngest child was abandoned at three months.

'We got him at the age of eight months and he's eleven months now. He's so fat. He can't even crawl. He just lies there. He came like a baby who was going to die any minute', observes Frances.

'What I notice with another child, who's two now, is that some days, he won't allow anybody to touch him. If the others accidentally push against him, he'll make a scene. Lab tests showed he has a bad bladder infection. He's also got oral thrush. I think there's a lot of things not right with him. When you put him down, he lies there till you pick him up again.

'Our only girl, Beauty, is three. She keeps her end up and screams if she can't have her way. When she came here, she wouldn't eat. She'd pick out the meat on the plate. And later on she wouldn't touch anything. She gave up porridge and then got dehydrated. In hospital, we said, "Doctor, we've got a problem." And it turned out she had oral thrush. She couldn't swallow and we didn't know it. When she came back from hospital she ate up all her food. But then two weeks ago she started a bad cough ...'

Beautiful Gate hasn't lost a child yet, but some of the children have been very sick at times.

'It's difficult to know how aware the children are of what's going on. When Beauty was hospitalised for a week, we told the others, "We must pray for Beauty." But I'm not sure what they took in. It's difficult to know whether any of them are distressed by whether they're wetting their beds or not, because sometimes they dirty the bed due to the diarrhoea and they all sweat a lot. Beds are often wet.'

At Beautiful Gate, plans have changed. Initially children were only going to be admitted if they came with a medical form stating their HIV-positive status. 'But,' says Frances, 'if you want to get the government subsidy [about £80 per institutionalised child per month], you have to have other kinds of children. You can't be specialised. We'll have to take another look at our constitution and change it. That requirement came through three months after we'd started.'

Beautiful Gate has survived so far on its links with Youth with a Mission, an international organisation that offers access to foreign volunteers and funds. Toby and Aukje also inspire donations by doing local press and radio interviews. Fundraising for an orphanage is relatively easy. Orphans are uncontroversial.

Frances has no idea how much it costs to run Beautiful Gate. The cost of an HIV-positive child at Nazareth House is about R2500 (£250) per month.

Foreign volunteers such as Harmke, the nursery school teacher, live on site. They give six to nine months of their time, and then return to their lives in Holland, America or Canada. There are also two childcare workers per shift. They live nearby and speak Xhosa to the children.

Beautiful Gate has just got a car. This will make an enormous difference. There will be more outings for the children. Harmke, an energetic young volunteer, really wants to get them out beyond the fence. Frances is more cautious,

> 'I'm not sure how our children would be received by the community. But we're going to do an experiment. There's a crèche just the other side of the fence. Harmke's going to see if our children can use the swings while their children are playing on them. We'll see how they react. We'd like our children to play with other kids, but if it's going to be traumatic for the children or for the staff or whatever … We'll see how it goes.'

So far, Harmke has tried three times to get the local school to have them over but has received no response. She'll keep trying.

Geographically, Beautiful Gate is in the middle of an impoverished community but the idea came from white outsiders, and it's run by them. With donations from near and far, they have achieved a level of material comfort for the children that is beyond that of their neighbours. The children have duvets, toys, furniture and curtains.

This can cause problems. 'We had some kids throwing stones and old shoes', sighs Frances. 'They broke some of the windows and the fence. I've seen them standing on the roofs, the other side of the fence, throwing rubbish over. Is it anger or vandalism? I'm not sure. We spoke to local leaders but we've had no feedback yet.'

To try to avoid a recurrence, and to try to manage the numbers of visitors who wander in at any time of the day to peer at the children like animals in a zoo, Frances is planning an open day. The public will be invited to look around and see what they are doing.

Beautiful Gate claims to provide AIDS education for the community. Certainly their childcare workers are local women and they are trained in order to do their job, but there is not yet much evidence of more extensive efforts. South African orphanages increasingly find that, to obtain public funding, they must provide some kind of educational service beyond their walls. They must change or close. The more dynamic now train volunteers in how to care for children, particularly those with HIV. They then send these people back into their communities with new skills and rubber gloves.

The Red Cross in Cape Town runs a course in how to provide basic nursing care for AIDS patients in their homes. The practical element of it is taught at Nazareth House. Jane knows this is good for trainees, but admits that sometimes they get under foot. 'We know we have to do more training out in the community, and I do believe in it,' she says reluctantly, 'but we haven't got the manpower. What worries me is what we do well – looking after the children – we may stop doing well.'

Routines get established quickly in institutions. Every day, the young Beautiful Gate residents are up, washed and dressed by eight in the morning. Whichever staff are around assist those who need help eating. After breakfast, the children receive their medication. And then the older ones attend nursery school from nine till 11.30.

Medicine time is popular. It's sweet, so the children gulp it down. Sometimes, if there are tears because someone has been told off, a member of staff will distract them by saying, 'Time for medicine. Who wants medicine?' And there will be a chorus of 'Me, me, me.'

Children in orphanages are hungry for affection. They rush to staff and visitors for hugs. They cling to adults' legs. They like to sit on adults and play with their watches or their earrings. If someone else seems to be getting a more central position in a hug, they shout, push and scramble in. As long as they are evenly distributed it is just about possible to have a child on each leg. When staff and visitors go home, they must gently peel them off.

'You see how when you come, they all stick up their hands to be picked up? Sometimes you'll have three children around you. How do you pick up three children?' asks Frances. 'You keep them around you like a hen, you know, just hold them like that. But sometimes that's not enough for them. They want to be picked up.'

The management try to discourage bonding between a child and a particular adult, but it's impossible to prevent it. Even Frances admits to having 'a special child'.

At Nazareth House they have a volunteer programme to try to find a special adult for each child; someone who might take the child out for weekends, shower it with affection and, who knows, maybe even foster or adopt it eventually.

'It's not working yet,' says Jane. 'but the aim is for every child to have somebody special.

'We don't usually allow people to take children out, if we don't know them. It's only when a volunteer's built up a close relation-ship with a child that I might suggest it. It takes time. You've got to know that person's going to be committed, because the child will cling to them. When they come back after a good weekend, they may cry.

'One of the volunteers who was hosting a child went off on holiday for three weeks at Christmas with her family and he pined for her. He was too little to understand that she was coming back and everybody said, "Maybe he shouldn't have that relationship", but the love he gets is so good when it's there. It's better than nothing. Hopefully one day they'll all have somebody like that.'

Back at Beautiful Gate, medicine time is over and the three older boys – Mandisi who's four, Bulelwa who's three and Mxolisi who's two and a half – head for their schoolroom. There are usually four in Harmke's class. Today, Beauty is in hospital, again. The other children don't seem to notice, until Harmke asks them directly, 'Who's missing? Who's usually sitting there?' and then they know it is Beauty.

Bulelwa likes to play in a tent. It is the only thing the three children do together. The rest of the time they play alongside, but not *with* each other. They sit at the same table but there is trouble if one of them touches another one's toy. They hardly ever look at each other unless they are competing for attention.

Harmke isn't surprised by the children's egoism. It's not odd at their age. In fact she is more concerned that Bulelwa is rather *too* unselfish. If another child is crying he gives his things to them.

Frances has noticed rivalry between Bulelwa, who arrived first, and Mandisi, the new boy who gets adult attention by being more confident and chatty. 'Mandisi's the one that's always in front and

Bulelwa resents him. He's been fighting a lot but Mandisi doesn't seem to be aware of it', observes Frances. When asked who his best friend is, Mandisi replies, 'Bulelwa.' Coming from another institution, he's used to lots of people. Bulelwa, on the other hand, had the attention of all the adults at Beautiful Gate to himself for a month before the other seven children arrived.

These children are behind in their development. Harmke thinks that it's more due to their past lack of stimulation than due to any physical cause. She thinks that Bulelwa is probably at least a year behind where he should be in terms of motor skills, knowing his colours and talking. He used to live on the street with his mum.

Frances watches the children.

'They play together and the bigger ones take care of the smaller ones but they do fight. It's strange how they all, if you are playing with a toy, will come and want that toy. That's how they behave here. They always want something that belongs to someone else.

'And I notice they're different from kids in an ordinary family home when they won't allow you to touch their things. If you sit next to them at table, you mustn't touch their food, their chair or the spoon they eat with. They're very possessive about their things. I think it's because they're from difficult backgrounds so it's security they're after. Even for the children who come from mummy. That mummy was sick and she had to look after a sick child. There may have been no communication beyond, "If you scream, I put you down and you stay there."'

Bulelwa's lack of words may also be due to linguistic confusion. Every day the children are exposed to English, Afrikaans and Xhosa. Harmke speaks English to them, with a Dutch accent. Bulelwa mixes Xhosa and English and rarely says a whole sentence in one language.

Mid-morning, Harmke has the children sitting round a low plastic table on little red plastic chairs. They have been playing with colourful play dough. Now it is time for a snack. She has them putting their hands together and singing their thanks before tucking into biscuits and juice. Then they move on to puzzles, picture books, tent games and putting on beads and hair bands. Beauty, particularly, likes jewellery and started a trend of wearing plastic hair bands across the forehead. Today, in her absence, Mxolisi is wearing his like that.

The children all play till lunchtime, sleep for a while, and then play until supper. If you arrive at Beautiful Gate just after lunch, there is not a sound. The children are sleeping and the staff are praying.

There is no doubt that the staff care deeply for the children at Beautiful Gate. But life in any orphanage is far from ideal. And new orphanages are an expensive way of tackling the AIDS orphan crisis. Even when orphanages are good at getting children into foster homes (which is difficult if they are HIV-positive), they can only ever help a fortunate few. To help larger numbers, efforts should probably be concentrated on educating pregnant women and supporting foster parents. HIV-positive mothers who understand that their babies have a good chance of surviving, because the majority of babies born to infected mothers do not contract the disease, are less likely to abandon them. Relatives or neighbours are more likely to foster an orphan if the state helps with the grocery bills and school fees.

Unaware of any of this, at frequent intervals throughout the day, Mandisi grins and does a cross between a thumbs up and a frantic hitchhiking gesture.

7
A Hundred Dollars for a Bull

A Social Worker's Story, Luweero District, Uganda

Bekunda Remigious lost his parents when he was a child. He bought himself an education by digging vegetables in the school garden and eventually won a degree in social work. Now he's married with a baby and running a project to help the swelling number of AIDS orphans in the Luweero district in central Uganda. Money from the Association François-Xavier Bagnoud (FXB), a Swiss–American foundation, enables him to kick-start small businesses for struggling foster parents and keep orphans in school by bartering furniture and roof repairs for free teaching. The hard currency goes a long way.

'The Luweero Triangle', in south central Uganda, was probably the worst affected area during the civil war that raged from 1979–86. Driving from the capital, Kampala, to Luweero, you see a burnt-out tank on the side of the road. Villagers point out the sites of mass graves. Orphans of the war are now adults, but a larger number of AIDS orphans have replaced them.

At 7.30am, mist hangs over the ground. The sunlight produces dazzling colours: red soil, lush green vegetation and blue sky. It's rush hour and the main road through the town of Luweero is lined with purposeful people walking to the fields and children in brightly-coloured school uniforms. At quieter times of the day, women walk with heavy bundles balanced on their heads and men push bicycles laden with branches of plantains, used to make *matoke*, the mushy local staple.

The FXB project, as it's known, started in the rural sub-county of Semuto in 1991 and has since been replicated in two other areas. It helps over 3,000 of the 8,000 orphans whom they have identified in the three sub-counties. Over half are AIDS orphans. Most of the villagers here are from the Baganda tribe who speak Luganda. Many live in remote clearings, along dirt tracks, almost hidden amid thick vegetation. A barely visible line of wire or a furrow running under the trees demarcates ownership of land. Some of their homes are round and thatched, others square and roofed with metal sheets.

FXB considers any child who has lost one or both parents to be an orphan, so many of the 'guardians' they help are actually widows who are struggling to look after their own children. Neil Monk, who did some research for FXB in Luweero in 1999, argues that the United Nations definition of an orphan (a child under 15 who has lost his mother or both parents) doesn't cover the situation in Luweero. Here, over half of the children who have lost their fathers, have absent mothers too. Children belong to the father's family, according to local customary law, so usually go to them after his death. Mothers are expected to go away and start a new family. Of the 732 orphans Monk surveyed, 63 per cent were paternal orphans, 16 per cent were maternal and 22 per cent had lost both parents.

FXB can't help all the orphans in Luweero, so they've devised a complex system to decide who qualifies for assistance. Bekunda explains it, 'First we told villagers and local leaders about the type of assistance that would be available. Then we asked them for a volunteer from each village, someone who is already looking after orphans, to devise parish orphan committees to identify the neediest orphans.'

In Uganda, a parish is an administrative rather than a religious entity, larger than a village but smaller than a sub-county. The parish orphan committee members bring a preliminary list of needy orphans to a meeting with local leaders and FXB staff where they decide together who should receive help. Making volunteers work alongside local leaders prevents either party choosing their family or friends.

'People used to try it on,' says Bekunda, 'but now nepotism has been reduced because it's a collective decision. This protects volunteers because they can tell disappointed guardians, "I have no power. Let me write your name down and I'll take it higher."'

Bekunda is confident that the system works. 'It's obvious who needs help most', he says. 'Decisions are based on how poor the guardian is, how sick they are and how many orphans they've got.' Meetings can grow heated, but he says that they usually reach a fair decision.

Perhaps; but it's not easy. There's a lot at stake. School fees paid for an orphan today could bear financial fruit for the whole family in future years.

'At a recent meeting, there were 40 orphans competing for five school places', says Bekunda. 'All were AIDS orphans, or soon will be. As it is, we just pick one child from each family and equal numbers of boys and girls. Sometimes guardians mind that we're educating an orphan while they cannot afford to educate their own children. But there's nothing we can do about this. We just encourage them by saying, "We've paid for this orphan's school lunches, so you must struggle and pay for lunch for the rest because it's unfair if your other four orphans go without." We accept it's a challenge and try to explain.'

As well as bringing orphans' names to the attention of the selection meeting, the volunteers on the parish orphans committee keep an eye out for orphans with problems. It's voluntary work, but as an incentive they get priority in getting a grant to start a small business. They are the crucial link between the community and FXB money.

Every three months, Bekunda gathers all the orphans and guardians they're helping together at a local school to see how they're coping. He deals with both sides: naughty orphans and abusive guardians.

'Guardians may say, "This orphan is trouble. He doesn't fetch water." Some orphans upset their guardians by getting pregnant or refusing to help with chores. But sometimes the orphan is refusing to go to school because the guardian is harassing his siblings. You ask both sides what is going on and then you advise them. They do respect my advice. Very few are stubborn.

'At each meeting, we write comments on the orphans' personal forms like, "This guardian was present. Orphan was not" or "Orphan dirty and miserable with jiggers [sand fleas that burrow under the skin of the feet]." The next time you see the child you might write, "Orphan very smart. Clean hair. Good shoes. Jiggers gone." It's nice to see progress and you thank the guardian at every opportunity so they go away happy.'

On many of the forms it clearly states the parents' cause of death as AIDS, rather than pneumonia or tuberculosis. There is little stigma around AIDS here. In schools, teachers talk openly about the AIDS orphans in their midst.

Since the Ugandan government introduced subsidised primary education for all in 1997, every child should, at least in theory, receive basic schooling. The government contributes around 500 shillings (about 20 pence) per child per term towards school fees and pays for textbooks, teachers' salaries and some school buildings. This still leaves parents shouldering about half the cost of their children's schooling. Many cannot afford even this, so lots of children, particularly orphans, are still denied an education.

This is where FXB steps in. The group barters free places for orphans at over 50 schools in exchange for classrooms, toilets, teachers' houses, head teachers' offices, desks, benches, typewriters, sewing machines, cooking equipment, bee hives, bicycles and even cows.

'We never give cash because the money might be diverted to other things', says Bekunda. 'Head teachers submit a budget each year and, after discussing and approving it, we take them to the shop, load the raw materials into the car and take them back to their school.'

Soon after becoming FXB's Boston-based Executive Director, Suzi Peel, a warm, former teacher with teenage daughters, visits Luweero to get a feel for the work she's now helping to fund. Everywhere she goes she receives a formal welcome and gushing gratitude. Bekunda acts as an intermediary between the foreign donor and the local people. He translates and tactfully deflects guardians' pleas for more money. He understands the donor's need for accountability and produces minutely detailed quarterly reports.

Bekunda takes Suzi to visit an array of schools and happy guardians. At the first stop, the St Mary of Rosary Kakinzi Primary School, 600 small children in bright pink uniforms sit in the sun waiting for the foreign visitor. Her organisation pays for many of them to be in school, so they wait respectfully. About 130 of them are orphans, of whom 70 are supported by FXB. The government has said that a child shouldn't be excluded from school just because her parents can't afford a uniform, but some head teachers insist anyway. At Kakinzi Primary, there are a few barefoot children without uniforms, conspicuous in the pink sea.

Before FXB came along, the school consisted of 30 kids doing lessons under a mango tree. Six years on, there are 14 teachers and proper classrooms, although it still looks like a building site. The school is a good example of co-operation between government, parents and a foreign donor. Parents brought the bricks, government supplied iron sheets for roofing and FXB donated desks, chairs and cement. All the children are benefiting, not just the orphans.

The acting headmaster, Robert Nkalubo, gives a 'Massage [sic] of appreciation' and asks for further assistance.

'We were orphans of war. Now there are orphans of AIDS. We have taken in three children who are sickly with HIV because they were lonely left at home. We've managed to get the children less dirty by concreting the floors to reduce dust levels. The roofs are on. Eventually we'll put in windows, but we need more chairs because our children can't write as nicely on the floor, and we're concerned about the quality of the drinking water we get from the dam because animals are using it.'

The children are impeccably behaved. They patiently observe the visiting *muzungu* (white) visitors while long, dull speeches are made on their behalf. Then a drum begins to beat, and a choir of schoolgirls in stripy socks shuffles rhythmically centre stage. They grin, sing and jiggle a cheerful greeting:

> It's our great pleasure, joy and excitement
> To welcome you, our dear visitors
> Our dear guest of honour, in your respect
> We are very happy to receive you all.
> FXB, you are welcome
> We are happy
> We are happy to receive you.

Suzi is presented with a collage of seeds and snail shells that thanks God for FXB.

Mary Mugerwa is the headmistress at Nalongo Primary School, the second stop on Suzi's itinerary. She seems irritated at having to entertain foreign visitors. Her school has a different atmosphere. Larger kids in blue uniforms push each other and chat while the headmistress tersely thanks FXB for sponsoring many of her pupils. A scrawny chicken walks by and pecks at the ground as four big girls and one little boy file in and recite a solemn poem:

> FXB, you are the mother
> You love us just like a real mother.
> What more could a mother do?
> FXB, I'm not ashamed to name you father
> I'm not grieved to call you mother,
> Because you've given me gold.
> Come what may I'm ready to study.
> With your support I will reach the top
> As long as FXB is.

Suzi addresses the kids,

'I'm very touched you're calling FXB your father and your mother and I will take that message back home. I'm grateful that there are people like Bekunda who are sort of your guardians if we are your parents. They let us know what you need. I want you to know we'll continue working for you and sending you help for a long time.'

Ugandan children singing that a donor agency is their mother – the gulf between rich north and poor south could hardly be more touchingly emphasised. But it's true. Financially, FXB *is* assuming responsibility for these kids.

In 1997, the project started offering a handful of scholarships so that the brightest orphans could go to secondary school. Under a tree in the grounds of Luweero Secondary School, Simon, Adolf and Paul sit in a row at the desk they've carried out to join Suzi and Bekunda. They're 13 or 14 years old and in their first year.

'These boys were lucky,' says Bekunda, 'because there could have been others who were better. In the whole sub-county, usually we pick only the four best ones, two girls and two boys. But this year, instead of taking four, I chose five, two girls and these three boys, because two got twelve points in their primary exams and the other had eleven. It was too difficult to choose between them, especially as Simon and Adolf have very sick mothers. So I somehow managed to spread the money to all three.'

He addresses the boys, 'How are you going to use the luck?' 'We are working so hard', say the boys in unison.

David joins the group. He is 15 and in his second year at the school. He is a brilliant pupil, as two scholarships attest. The school is now paying for two terms of fees and Bekunda supplies books for him. David is sharp. He pretends to be laid back, but he watches foreign visitors intently. He has aspirations. He wants to be a politician.

Bekunda asks the orphans if they need anything. For starters, David wants more than the four years of schooling that FXB is providing. He asks Suzi to pay for the full six years of secondary school so that he can go to university. Bekunda interjects and tells him that it's not possible because there are so many orphans. It's a matter of balancing how many years of education FXB can provide against how many children should be reached.

David complains that his bike ride to school takes 50 minutes and leaves him too tired to study when he gets home. Paul, too, has a long commute. Every day he walks six kilometres to the main road where he can board a minibus taxi for another 14 kilometres to school.

'I can see it's a problem', agrees Bekunda. 'At this school we have students who are boarders competing with people who have to cycle or walk far and, on reaching home, have to look for firewood. It's not fair. We'll review our budget and if we find we have the money we'll try and help you to stay nearer school.'

'Is that the solution you want?' asks Suzi.

'Yes', say all the boys, grinning.

Adolf, the most confident of the three smaller boys, asks for a chemistry textbook.

'OK, that one's easier', says Bekunda. 'You must identify the textbook you want, and the price, and tell me next time I come here. I'll buy one copy and you can share it.'

'It's 8000 shillings [about £3.20]', pipes up Adolf immediately.

The boys complain that they have only one uniform each and they get sweaty travelling to school. Bekunda reminds them of the original meeting they had when he told their guardians what FXB would donate and what the guardians must strive to provide. Uniforms fell into the latter category.

'But our guardians are poor', says Adolf matter-of-factly.

Suzi tells them, 'An important lesson is to learn to ask. Sometimes the other person will say, "Sorry, it's not possible." But, sometimes, they'll say, "OK."'

It's a lesson that David and Adolf have mastered.

'Instead of boarding, could we rent a place near school?' suggests David.

'Do you feel you could stay in one room? Do you know how to cook? Find out how much the rent would be', says Bekunda.

David nods, satisfied, and then says wistfully, 'I'd also like to visit America.'

'Now that's more like wishful thinking', replies Bekunda.

Bekunda is a role model for them. They know he was an orphan and they're ambitious like he was.

Leaving the scholars, Bekunda say, 'Yes, I see myself in those boys.' For them, he'll squeeze five scholarships out of four and locate textbooks and rented accommodation, but he'll also give them tough advice, 'Know that life isn't easy now. It'll get easier in 10–15 years time.'

The other half of the FXB project aims to uplift orphans by helping their guardians earn more money. The whole family benefits. These guardians have, on average, taken in five extra orphans on top of their own children. FXB has given over 800 of them a grant of US$100 to start a small business. Guardians have opened shops with the money. They've taken up tailoring, photography, brewing, bee-keeping, brick-making, growing cash crops such as coffee and rearing livestock such as cows and chickens. But by far the simplest and most popular option has proved to be bull-rearing.

'Guardians decide what they want to do. They already know what goes and what doesn't and they get ideas from others who've already embarked on it. We know there's a big market for meat because, in our culture, people eat meat every weekend. Guardians know they can get a bull or cow from markets where there are people who have thousands and so perhaps haven't fed them well. Once they get it home, it fattens up quickly on banana peels and can be sold for a profit within nine months.

'Once a guardian's application has been approved at the selection meeting, and they've been trained, we go with them to the market. We shop with them the first time, and then they're on their own.'

When the project started, $100 was worth 100,000 shillings, which bought a bull. Due to inflation, $100 is now worth 150,000 shillings which means guardians can afford a cow, which is considered a better investment because it produces milk and calves.

'It's not a loan', says Bekunda. 'We don't expect them to pay it back because we're dealing with the poorest of the poor and they're simply not credit-worthy. And a grant's a lot simpler to administer than credit systems, although obviously less sustainable because the money isn't coming back into the pot.'

Novice entrepreneurs in these types of projects often fail to make a profit because they haven't grasped basic business skills. However, about 80 per cent of the FXB guardians' businesses succeed. It helps that they are given items in kind and training so that they understand that, for example, eating the bull will cause the business to collapse. Those who fail through misfortune are bailed out from the FXB emergency fund. Those who fail through bad management are not.

Margret Higenyi, 58, a widow with six children, got her first bull in 1996. She sold it and bought three more, but one night they were stolen. The FXB emergency fund paid her transport costs to trace and recover the bulls. The culprit was apprehended. She later sold two of the bulls and used the proceeds to buy a cow and school uniforms and shoes for the children. The fund is also used for crises such as a missing orphan or the collapse of a guardian's house.

Bekunda describes Winnie Tumuheirwe as old. She's 50. She lives in a village called Kiiya with her nine orphaned grandchildren. In 1992, a $100 grant bought her six black and white goats. Now she has five goats, plus two majestic, big-horned bulls. Piles of branches heavy with bananas lie outside her house. They'll be sold too.

Winnie says, 'These are my grandchildren. Six are my son's children. He died in 1989 and his wife disappeared during the war. She probably died too. I had three children. The eldest became mentally disturbed. He's over there, hiding behind that bush. My daughter got married but her husband died, so I have three of her children too. I was already taking care of the children before my son died but in those days I was still confident because my son was supporting us. The youngest child was one week old when it was left to me. The oldest one, Bernard, is 20 now.

'Our local leaders called us to a meeting and we each said how many orphans we look after. We were given assistance depending on this. Bernard was one of the first to get FXB assistance while he was in primary. Now he's in secondary. Later, we found out that we could go to the office for help with application forms for projects to make money. Unfortunately I was not among the first to receive this, but I was patient and later I was informed that my application had been accepted. I was given an appointment to discuss the activity I'd requested. Then I was told that goats had been found for me. I was given three old ones and three young ones. I got the idea because when I was young, my parents looked after goats. The goats helped them look after me.

'I tried my best to look after the six goats but three died after a year. The three remaining ones were the young ones, luckily, and they each produced twice, so then I had nine goats. The FXB social worker advised me that since my goats had become many, and in case a disease should kill them all, I should save a few and sell the others to get money and buy cows. I sold four goats, got 70,000 shillings [about £28] and bought a bull. After a year, I sold the bull and got 270,000 shillings [about £108]. Some of this went on school fees but the rest paid for three more bulls, one of which I've sold since then, leaving me with five goats and two bulls.'

She pauses, and then asks, 'Can FXB give me credit because my bull is not ready for selling but I need money to send Bernard to university?'

Bekunda gently explains that FXB only gives one-off grants of $100, never credit.

In Ngogolo village, a slightly more built-up area, Beatrice Byanyima, 35, who lost her husband in 1994, has opened a hair salon with her $100 grant. Bekunda is proud of her. He describes her business, which has diversified into a restaurant and hotel, in glowing terms. However, in the middle of a Tuesday morning, the place is shut up, and when she finally appears, she looks downcast. She's struggling to pay school fees for her eight children. Her profits are too small.

Beatrice is pretty. She wears a turquoise dress with puffed-up sleeves and a pink scarf, wrapped around her head, turban-style. Little tassels shake as she talks.

'A year after my husband died, FXB came to me with assistance and I started the hair salon. I had nothing to do except to work. It's good in the two holiday seasons from June to August and from September to January with about 20 customers a day, but out of season, it's a struggle, you may get one or two people a day. I opened a hotel and restaurant next to the salon but I don't get many customers. It's slow right now. Today I was working in my *shamba* [plot]. During the holidays the children work there. I work hard. You can't do anything without money.

'Now, some of the children are in secondary and the money is not enough. I use all my savings to send them to a good school. I am suffering with them. I'm the auntie, the father, the grandmother, everything. My oldest is 17 and my youngest is very sick.'

After leaving Beatrice, Bekunda admits that the guardians and orphans' problems sometimes feel overwhelming.

'I work many weekends. It's tiring. Guardians come to me even when I'm not in the office and say, "The orphan was defiled." It's stressful at times because I can empathise when they come crying, "I don't have school fees." But I have a limited budget. All I can do is encourage them not to lose hope and just do what they can. We have so many applications, we cannot get through them, but we keep promising, "You may be assisted in the future."'

FXB is an intriguing organisation. When asked what its criteria for funding projects are, Suzi replies, 'The only way to answer that is to tell the founder, Countess Albina du Boisrouvray's story. There are no other criteria.' And she proceeds to tell her boss's life story like a fairy tale.

'Albina was the only child of a French count. Her mother was the daughter of an enormously wealthy family who owned silver and tin mines in Bolivia. She went to a Swiss finishing school and fell in love with her dashing ski instructor, Bruno Bagnoud. He was a rescue helicopter pilot in the Swiss Alps. They had a blond, blue-eyed, baby boy called François-Xavier Bagnoud who looked like *Le Petit Prince* [the hero of a classic children's book by Antoine De Saint-Exupéry]. He became a helicopter pilot and did Alps rescue work like his father. In 1986, he was accompanying the Paris–Dakar rally through Mali. His helicopter, like the narrator in *Le Petit Prince*, crashed over the desert. He and two passengers were killed. Nobody knows why. He was 24.

'Albina went into shock. This was her only child. As she came through her grief she decided to take everything that would have been his inheritance and sell it. The art collection, jewellery, castles and a film business endowed a foundation to the tune of about $100 million. Albina decided to use it for children in need and so to keep her son's name alive.'

FXB now operates out of Boston, New York and Geneva. Its budget of US$5 million a year supports work with street kids in Uruguay, HIV-positive babies in Colombia, Thailand and India, prostitutes in Myanmar and Thailand, widows and children in Rwanda and AIDS orphans in Uganda, South Africa, Zambia and Zimbabwe.

'Every FXB project is different,' says Suzi, 'but most are concerned with children and HIV, and our focus has become AIDS orphans. Albina's philosophy is to check where people are falling through safety nets. It's often children, and among children, it's often orphans, and among orphans it's often AIDS orphans.'

Albina cuts an unlikely figure. Everyone in the small circle who attends AIDS conferences knows her because she's been involved for over a decade and because she's more glamorous and French than the average NGO worker. She pouts, flicks her hair and tosses a brightly-coloured scarf over a shoulder while delivering a passionate speech about AIDS orphans.

She wants to persuade the world's richest companies and individuals, the top few hundred of whom are listed annually by *Forbes* magazine, to give, once off, 2 per cent of their wealth to children's projects, particularly those that target street children and AIDS orphans. If she pulls it off, this cause would receive an endowment of US$40 billion, yielding US$2 billion a year. It's part of her vision of creating 'a global village' to help AIDS orphans around the world.

Her organisation, FXB, is a small, whimsical outfit, but it has a flexibility and straightforwardness that's lacking in the vast bureaucracies of the United Nations Children's Fund (UNICEF) or the United States Agency for International Development (USAID), the big players in the field of helping AIDS orphans.

The FXB project in Luweero is simple and effective. It gives an elderly guardian or a widow a manageable source of income – a cow is easy to understand – and gives four extra years of schooling to clever children. It tries to cultivate leaders by assisting a few talented scholars, but also spreads money thinner and wider through guardians' businesses and by helping all the children at a few dozen primary schools. It isn't sustainable indefinitely, but, at the moment, many guardians and orphans benefit.

The project is in safe hands with Bekunda. An annual budget of US$140,000 goes a long way in Luweero. Whether or not a project works, and whether the participants stay motivated, depends on the project's leader. Bekunda is firm and compassionate. He keeps money coming in from Albina's World, and constantly boosts the morale of the guardians and orphans he is trying to support.

In Bekunda's little office in Butuntumula village, one wall is covered by a poster of the dashing young European, in whose memory some of Albina's personal fortune has been donated to poor families in rural Uganda. It seems incongruous, but it's unlikely that any of the guardians who have received US$100 for a bull ponder for long about the source of their good fortune.

Section III

International Involvement

8
Foreign Aid or Interference?

United Nations Children's Fund (UNICEF), Lusaka, Zambia

Peter McDermott is the country representative for the United Nation's Children's Fund (UNICEF), the largest of the 13 United Nations (UN) agencies operating in Lusaka, the capital of Zambia. Using the promise of more donor funding as a carrot, he's pushing politicians to be accountable. This is not always easy.

'They call me the guerrilla bureaucrat,' he says, 'because if there's a way of getting around the system, I will. You have to manipulate to get things done.'

'My job's to provide leadership in UNICEF-Zambia, and through that to Zambia's government and non-governmental organisations (NGOs), to mobilise commitment and action to ensure children get due recognition and resources.' He pauses, grins and adds, 'And agitate – infiltrate and agitate!'

He guffaws. He spends a lot of his time trying to influence people and clearly enjoys it.

The Zambian government was slow to get to grips with AIDS.

'The government infrastructure here is weak', he explains. 'Zambia was a single party, socialist state until 1991. There was only one mechanism for dealing with things (through central government) and by the late '80s it had virtually collapsed and there was no service provision at all. It's still almost non-existent.

'Since then, much has been done in terms of privatising the economy and opening things up, but because for that 10–15 years when the pandemic was beginning to take a hold, there was such a weak, centralised infrastructure, it meant that Zambia didn't develop a tradition of NGOs and churches to handle the issues. Lots of NGOs have sprung up in recent years, but they're small and inexperienced.

'The current government is trying to put up new structures like an AIDS Council to produce a national strategy and co-ordinate

AIDS activities, but they have few resources and a huge debt burden.'

Committee Room Four in the Zambian parliament buildings is dark and has noisy air conditioning and damp patches on the wall. Four Members of Parliament sit at one end of a big table. Peter sits at the other. The MPs are all Big Men, both literally and metaphorically. The other half of the committee is away at funerals or 'on parliamentary business in Kenya'.

Parliament's not in session, but Peter has been invited to make a presentation to this parliamentary sub-committee, which deals with health and welfare matters. Peter's goal today is to persuade them to get parliament to declare AIDS a national disaster and hold a special parliamentary session on it.

It's almost like a game. Permission to speak is always sought through the Chairman. Peter throws the ball firmly into the MPs' court. 'If the government's new AIDS Council produces a national framework for AIDS activities,' he tells them, 'the donor community in Zambia will produce significantly more funding'. He tells the MPs about a meeting he's had that morning with a donor. If they get their act together, this source alone will donate over US$1 million to the new AIDS Council's work.

It's strange watching a foreigner inform a group of MPs what's happening in their country. Donor organisations usually have bigger computers, more researchers and better databases than lawmakers do in developing countries. Peter reels off statistics and urges the MPs to stand up and lead other nations in the fight against AIDS. When he's finished, one of the MPs asks plaintively, 'But what can parliament do when we don't have any money?'

Peter replies that declaring AIDS a national disaster, as President Daniel arap Moi in Kenya and President Robert Mugabe in Zimbabwe have recently done, costs nothing but helps break the silence around the disease and signals that the government is taking the situation seriously. And if they commit whatever small sums are available in the government coffers and pledge future resources to tackling poverty and AIDS, then donors would match these amounts tenfold.

Genuinely puzzled, an MP asks Peter, 'Why's the government been slow to respond?'

The MPs discuss bringing a private member's motion to debate AIDS in parliament but they think a preliminary briefing session would be needed, because, as the Chairman points out, some MPs don't know how AIDS is transmitted.

As the proceedings draw to a close, the Chairman reminds Peter, in a roundabout way, of an earlier offer by UNICEF to sponsor MPs on a study tour to another country badly affected by HIV/AIDS. Peter agrees to make good this promise, but asks that a single request from the group of MPs be made to his office. He doesn't want individual MPs coming to him asking for trips. The committee members become animated and toy with the idea of a study tour to Uganda, Botswana, or maybe, Thailand ...

Driving back from parliament, Peter's pleased with how it went. 'I wondered when they'd get round to asking for the study tour!' he laughs. The formality of the meeting disguised the fact that he knows these men quite well, having, on other occasions, shared beers with them.

> 'You have to ask for lots of things. Then you'll get some of them. If you ask for one thing and you don't get it, you're disappointed. Zambians are very open. If they feel you have Zambia's interests at heart, they'll listen to what you have to say. It's all down to trust.' He understands the rules of the game. 'They want certain things from us. We want certain things from them. Is there a negotiating position?'

The next day, Peter, a few of his colleagues and a senior Zambian AIDS official are sitting conspiratorially round the table in Peter's office. They're talking tactics for the monthly AIDS meeting of all Lusaka-based UN and other donor agencies later in the day. No high-level government people have agreed to attend. Consequently, the meeting's agenda – to discuss how to push ahead with the government's response to AIDS – looks fairly pointless. Peter decides to have one last go at persuading the politicians along.

He dials a number and to his surprise he gets straight through to the Cabinet Secretary. The team round the table goes quiet, watching Peter operate. 'Good morning, *Sir!*' says Peter breezily. He uses a mixture of exaggerated deference and the tone one might use with an old school chum. 'Wouldn't want government to miss out on donor funding, your Excellency ... You know my loyalty to government ...' He's pressing all the right buttons. It works. The man agrees to show up. Peter comes back to the table, grinning. His colleagues are amazed.

A few minutes later, a top-ranking civil servant, who had previously been unavailable to attend, calls. It now appears that he can come. He can't miss it, if his superior's going to be there. 'You've been ignoring me', says Peter playfully, 'I must have upset you!' It's said with such a light touch, he gets away with it. 'Delighted you can come ... We're honoured', says Peter. His grin gets even bigger.

The new AIDS Council needs office space. The team round the table wants to sort this out soon because otherwise the government's AIDS work will be held up even longer. They consider which donors might be willing to buy a building quickly. There are also rumours that someone in government is trying to make money out of the property deal. The team discusses how to thwart such shenanigans before they start without actually saying, 'The donors will only buy *this* particular building.' If they did that, and things went wrong with the AIDS Council, the politicians might distance themselves from its work by saying it's 'owned' by the donor community.

No government likes foreigners telling it what to do. Words such as 'partnership' and 'alliance' don't eradicate the sometimes mutually suspicious relationship between benefactor and beneficiary. Being dependent on foreign money is uncomfortable. Money's welcome, interference is not. A Zambian NGO worker observes,

> 'Sometimes in our country we only respond to things when there's been donor pressure. I think most of the institutions of authority feel belittled if they're told, "This is the right thing to do." It's pride. If they initiate it, then that's good, but they feel that anything coming from another sector is like a command. They may do it much later when people have forgotten that the idea came out of a workshop run by outsiders.'

There's an hour left until the donor meeting; just time for UNICEF staff to reshuffle the agenda and ring round important ambassadors to get them to attend in person, now that they know there are going to be government people worth lobbying there.

Thirty suited men and a sprinkling of women pack into the boardroom in the UN building. Chairs are two deep around a big oval table. This group of people, from the world's richer countries, represents the source of about 90 per cent of Zambia's money for AIDS control.

One of the donor organisations has been causing waves. It recently offered funding to help build up the country's infrastructure but the Zambian government rejected the proposal because it involved too many expatriate consultants. Stiff letters were fired off both ways. Peter is exasperated. Such unsubtle, unilateral action creates tensions and makes life harder for everyone else. Arrogance provokes resistance. Tactful suggestions, discreet monitoring of expenditure and co-operation amongst the donor community is more likely to get money spent constructively.

The two Lusaka-based UN Joint Programme on HIV/AIDS (UNAIDS) representatives, whose job is to co-ordinate the UN's response to the epidemic, present a spreadsheet of which donors are funding what areas of AIDS work in Zambia. They encourage anyone with money to spend on AIDS to put it into the new AIDS Council or projects targeting farm workers, soldiers, street children, religious groups or girl guides and boy scouts.

Suddenly, the Cabinet Secretary makes a grand entrance. The speaker falls silent. Everyone stands. The Cabinet Secretary sits at the head of the table and reads out his speech, a potted history of the government's action on AIDS. It doesn't take very long. He doesn't dwell on the fact that two months after the Cabinet formed the AIDS Council, it still hasn't met, chosen a chairperson or even defined its goals.

He ends his speech with an appeal for funds. His colleague leads the clapping and then says a few words beginning, 'It is procedurally difficult for me to speak after my boss, who so brilliantly presented the issues …'

One of the donors tells the Cabinet Secretary, 'Money's burning in my hand. I haven't been able to spend it on AIDS here. I've been waiting for a strategic framework from your government.'

Another asks if there will be a similar Council for co-ordinating a national response to orphans. The Cabinet Secretary replies, 'The issue of orphans is extremely pressing. We have a number of NGOs dealing with it. I can't just talk and talk like … I was going to say like the UN.' People laugh politely. Peter recommends setting up a steering committee for orphans and vulnerable children, under the new AIDS Council, rather than another new inter-ministerial structure.

In the absence of government co-ordination, Peter is thinking of setting up a monthly forum on orphans, possibly co-chaired with a non-governmental umbrella organisation, Children in Need, itself funded by UNICEF. It is important for locals to feel that they 'own' the project. But there are pitfalls. When government bureaucracy takes over initiatives, inertia sets in. Peter wonders if it might be possible to keep such a committee half in, and half out of, the new AIDS Council's jurisdiction.

After the meeting, Peter is buoyant. It went well. It's satisfying pinning politicians down. He plans to write and thank the Cabinet Secretary and confirm what they heard him say. 'We look forward to more action on the AIDS Council in the next fortnight', he'll write. It's taken months to get the man to this point. It's another small triumph.

'Today's donor meeting was classic', says Peter. 'We had a problem – things not going fast enough – but we may have turned it around by just being fortuitous with the Cabinet Secretary picking up his phone.

'We've also wanted a parliamentary debate on AIDS for a long time, and in yesterday's parliamentary sub-committee meeting we planted the seeds. I don't know yet if what occurred in these two meetings represents a real shift forward. We seized the opportunities, but we may look back in six weeks and say, "Nothing happened." So we have to keep pushing, every day, at every level and not just at national government.'

Peter's a tall Englishman, with a confident stride, a firm handshake and seemingly unshakeable optimism. He's worked for UNICEF for 15 years and lived in Zambia for the past two. Before that he worked in war zones. 'Wherever there was a conflict, my job was to go in and make sure UNICEF had a presence and got assistance in. You name a war zone between 1991 and 1998 ... We lost a lot of staff.'

Peter points to a big black and white photo on his office wall. It shows a young man with his back to the camera. He's wearing a UN shirt and supervising people loading food into a four-by-four. He was working for Peter in Mogadishu, the capital of Somalia. UNICEF was trying to get food to starving Somalis in the midst of a chaotic civil war. He was killed the day after the photo was taken. He was 26.

'I miss the adrenaline of working in a war zone. It was very immediate. You can see the result of your actions much quicker, but you also see the raw depths of humanity. In theory, coming to Lusaka was meant to be a quiet posting and a return to development work for me, but the amount of death here is really on a par with, and in many cases much worse than, many emergencies. And it's been going on for 15 years. Apart from Rwanda and Mogadishu, I've rarely seen this level of death on a daily basis. The difference is it's not in your face here. It's behind closed doors and there isn't the anger or outcry or moral disgust at what's going on.

'Zambia's never been at war. It was the third richest African country at independence, 35 years ago. But now, you look at the infant mortality rate and nutrition rate, and they're equivalent to maybe Afghanistan or Somalia, and you ask yourself why in a country so well endowed – with resources, land, lovely people and peace – are people so poor? Why are things so bad?'

He answers himself, 'Issues of governance, allocation of resources, strategic choices.'

In other words, the Zambian government's messed up. Zambia is one of the few countries (of those where data's been available) whose Human Development Index value (a measure of life expectancy, access to education and economic growth) is lower now than it was in 1975. Zambia now spends more servicing its US$7 billion external debt than on health and education combined. The country was not aided by donors who were only too willing to fund things that were not in the interest of the majority of Zambians. AIDS has made things much worse. There's so much to be done. Peter works at running pace, but still feels, 'We have to find ways of doing more, quicker. You always feel you're not doing enough.'

At the end of a long day, Peter sips a glass of wine in a hotel bar with lots of fountains and elaborately thatched tables. He looks tired, but has another function to go on to later, which is why he's carrying a fancy floral arrangement for a diplomat's wife.

'You do get bad days, you know, when the bureaucracy gets you down. You screw up. You get reprimanded for things. You push the envelope too far. It backfires. Fortunately I have far more good days than bad days. I've been overseas so long, that wherever I am, I feel comfortable. It should be a three-year posting here but I'll try and do a fourth if I can. I like it here, and it's only after a while that you get effective.'

UNICEF is a billion-dollar organisation, with 6,000 staff working in over 140 countries. It relies on charitable donations for nearly a third of its US$960 million annual budget. Peter is keen to stress that UNICEF is not a donor agency, despite the fact that they fund government and NGO activities.

'We're a UN agency,' he says, emphatically, 'that supports national governments' efforts. We're not like a British or a US government, which donates money direct to the Zambian government. The international community makes money available to Zambia for children's activities and entrusts UNICEF to plan and manage it with the Zambian government. We don't just hand the money over. We have it in trust to make sure it's used for the purposes it's given. The governments who give us money set out what our goals are and our strategy to achieve them.'

This is why UNICEF cannot distribute condoms. The US government and the Vatican dislike the idea of a children's organisation handing them out.

'The implementation of UNICEF's strategy at country level is negotiated between the local UNICEF office and the government. Governments of developing countries are much less compliant nowadays. Many years ago, UNICEF might have been more authoritative. Nowadays, there's genuine negotiation with governments on how to operate together. Our role varies depending on how strong or weak the government is. In South Africa, for instance, UNICEF assists policy-making but it's a very limited role, because there's plenty of local expertise there. In other countries, especially emergency countries like Somalia where there is no government, UNICEF is immunising children and providing water and schools like an NGO.'

UNICEF-Zambia has 51 staff including 13 expatriates plus a handful of consultants on short-term contracts. Their budget between 1997 and 2001 was about US$12 million a year, 80 per cent of which was committed to programmes with the government.

Peter starts every Monday morning with a 'stand-up' meeting. His team of managers report progress and problems in the five departments: water, child protection, education, health and office management. An outsider might have little idea of what they're talking about because they speak in acronyms. They talk about 'OVCs' (orphans and vulnerable children) and 'CEDCs' (children in especially difficult circumstances), PPAs (project plan of action) and LTAs (long-term agreements).

One of Peter's managers looks very ill. He's distracted, and says he will attend a meeting, if he's well enough. A competent deputy is covering for him. AIDS is a problem inside the office as well as outside. In 1999, there were two staff deaths and one staff member's spouse and another's child also died. Four hundred days were lost due to illness, compared to 166 the year before. Peter has managed to wangle cheap anti-retroviral drugs as a perk for HIV-positive staff.

> 'It's not a UN-wide policy. Zambia's the only country doing this at the moment. I set it up because I believe you can't fight a battle if your troops are sick. And also you need the confidence of your staff that you're looking after them and not just some other group. It wasn't easy to work the UN bureaucracy on this. The reason I got away with it is probably because a lot of people don't know I'm doing it.'

Another day, Peter joins the child protection team's departmental meeting. Their job is to lobby the Zambian government to review all child-related legislation, reform the juvenile justice system, set up a committee on orphans to produce a national orphan strategy, improve social services for street children and establish minimum standards for orphanages.

The staff are mostly quite junior and seem slightly intimidated by having their work come under Peter's scrutiny. The meeting gets bogged down on the first thing discussed, a strategy on child abuse. The young man responsible for this area looks stressed. There's too much for him to do. Child abuse is clearly an issue UNICEF should be dealing with, but, in the absence of relevant statistics, research or a national strategy, he doesn't know where to start. Peter's probing questions make him defensive. Eventually, Peter's suggests he commission someone to do the necessary research before a strategy can be drafted.

> 'Our job,' he explains later, 'is to manage the process of completion, so products are done on time, but experts and NGOs are contracted in to do the implementation. It's a real balancing act because at the end of the day, it's not about us. The issue is

how to get Zambia – government, churches, NGOs, Zambian people – to do more for themselves with or without us. We have to try and get people to take on the responsibility that they have. If they don't have the resources or technical skills, in some cases, we can provide them. You always have to be careful, because sometimes it's easier to grab it and do it yourself. You fall into this trap all the time. But that's not why we're here.

'Yes, I know I'm a doer', he says, and laughs. 'My staff get very tired.'

If you were lazy and ineffectual, you'd be very aware of your inadequacies in Peter's presence. He sets deadlines. He stops staff in the corridor to ask if they've made a particular phone call yet. He gets results.

UNICEF-Zambia excels at gathering and sharing information. In 1998, UNICEF paid a couple of consultants to spend three weeks in Zambia doing a 'Polaroid snapshot' of research on the orphan situation. A year later, 20 consultants spent four months working on a much bigger research project resulting in a 400-page report, *Orphans and Vulnerable Children: A situation analysis, Zambia 1999.* It's a dry read but probably the most comprehensive study on AIDS orphans from anywhere in sub-Saharan Africa. UNICEF-Zambia publicised the report, even producing it on CD-ROM, so that people can cut and paste bits into their proposals or articles.

The research revealed that 44 per cent of Zambian households are looking after orphans and argued that we shouldn't distinguish between orphans and other needy children because, in Zambia, at least, orphans aren't being discriminated against. It's poverty and not AIDS that is the overriding determinant of whether a child is adequately cared for or not. Orphans are often materially deprived, but not much more so than children whose parents are alive. This is counter-intuitive. Most researchers assume that AIDS orphans would have formed a new underclass, worse off than the poorest Zambians and perhaps ostracised into the bargain. But this is not the case. In fact, the report warned that NGO workers, by going into villages and asking to count AIDS orphans, might unwittingly have introduced a stigma where there was none before.

But the research is only the starting point.

'Despite now having all this data,' says Peter, 'the orphan response is still fragmented because, in the absence of a national strategy, donors have come up with slightly different ideas on where they think funding should go. Some say, "We've got the money. We'll do our own thing and bring in expatriate consultants to do it." They don't always get the community genuinely involved and aren't bothered whether they're working within a national government co-ordinated framework or not. They just want to spend the money and show a result. Then after two years or so, they leave and it's hard to know what's left behind after them. There's a real risk that too much money, badly placed, could undermine communities' efforts, if they become dependent on donors.

'The other type of donor sees their role as strengthening local communities to take charge of their own responsibilities towards orphans and ultimately coping without external funding. Their approach tends to be more slow and meticulous, sometimes to the point of being ponderous. There's a tension between the need to have an urgent response of huge proportions because of the scale of the problem, and being committed to a community response. There are no answers I'm afraid.

'I think UNICEF's job is to highlight the pros and cons of the different approaches. If we have a position it's that the solution has to be with the communities, but we can play a catalytic role to help them.

'One of the big lessons we learnt from our 1999 research was how to scale up good projects. The answer is not to think that you can make good, small projects bigger. What we need is thousands more good, small projects; a mass of projects, not one massive project. Activities at grass roots level will always be *ad hoc*, and I think they have to be. We shouldn't try to control them.'

Peter acts as a traffic controller for outsiders interested in giving money to Zambia. They come for advice and he describes Zambia's national response to date. 'The UN has by stealth assumed the co-ordinating role,' explains Peter, 'but we want government to take it on. As more money has been given to Zambia over the last two years, it's increasingly important that activities are co-ordinated nationally to avoid duplication and to discourage donors funding outside a national strategy.' Peter thinks government must at least try to lay 'railway lines' and get agencies working within them.

Funders have a dilemma: how to give money flexibly, so that it may be used to best effect, but ensure that it isn't stolen. Where corruption is a problem, donors tend to demand transparency. Peter advises potential donors that they should be more concerned about accountability. Major projects must have an external audit after 18 months. 'At the end of the day we want an AIDS programme that works', he says.

Peter exerts no pressure, but undoubtedly influences how donors spend their money. It's time-consuming, but increases the likelihood that money given by foreigners, with very little idea of what's going on in Zambia, will be put to best use.

Lots of people want a piece of his time, so he has one meeting after another, running approximately 20 minutes late, throughout the day. He talks fast. You can see him working through the bullet points of an agenda in his mind and when someone's time is up, he starts looking at his watch. Even so, his visitors invariably say, 'Just one more question', and ask two more, although the next person's waiting outside to tap into Peter's expertise.

A lot of vital time was wasted during the 1990s. The international community virtually ignored the issue of AIDS orphans between 1991–97. 'The fear was that it was a charity issue', Susan Hunter (who has worked for both UNICEF and the United States Agency for International Development) told the audience at the first conference on AIDS orphans to be held in South Africa in 1998. 'There was no way the North could support all the orphans in the South, so none of the donors or international agencies really wanted to put effort into it. They decided instead to put effort into AIDS prevention ... There was a time when we believed that we could stop this epidemic.'

Things have moved on since 1999. Peter observes,

'The sheer numbers of orphans now are something that's so morally reprehensible that people are taking note. Children inspire guilt. We've tried to separate HIV (the sexually transmitted disease) from its impact (the orphans), because everyone can rally around children. UNICEF can put children in the front line of a debate, because it's believed they're apolitical.

'We woke up the World Bank and other donors by holding up a mirror and saying, "Look, you've put $20 billion of development assistance into Africa over the last 10–15 years and all of a sudden the goals you've set yourselves and the gains your investment has achieved, such as reducing infant mortality and getting healthy immunised children into schools, are being eroded by AIDS. So unless you want your $20 billion thrown out the window we'd better start addressing the problem."'

In January 2000, the UN Security Council debated the impact of AIDS in Africa. It was the first time they'd discussed a health issue as a threat to peace and security. Kofi Annan, the UN Secretary-General, said that by overwhelming the continent's health services, by creating millions of orphans and by decimating health workers and teachers, AIDS threatens political stability. Given that many African countries are already unstable, AIDS could mean the difference between peace and civil war.

Peter says,

'Nobody was thinking through what the implications of this epidemic were for the stability of states, having hundreds of thousands of destitute people, at a time when the US and others were feeling, "We don't need any more problems in the world. We don't want to have to come in and bail them out."'

In 1996, recognising that diseases like the HIV virus don't respect national borders, the US government started examining its policy on AIDS in Africa. In 1998, 57 million Americans went overseas for business or pleasure, twice the number a decade before. A million immigrants and refugees enter the US legally every year and several hundred thousand more slip in without papers. As the epidemic increases instability in developing countries, more US forces will be expensively and riskily deployed on humanitarian and peacekeeping operations.

Consequently, the US government donated US$80 million to AIDS activities in sub-Saharan Africa in 1999, which rose to US$120 million in 2000, four times as much as the next donor and twice as much as the World Bank. This sounds a lot but UNAIDS estimates that US$3 billion is required annually for HIV prevention and care globally. Current resources available are about a tenth of this.

Finally, the world's media got interested in covering the story of AIDS in Africa. 'Only then did it became a political issue', observes Peter. 'And many groups – NGOs, church groups, the UN, donors, governments – suddenly came together and realised, "We can actually do something." Before that, fatalism was everywhere.'

One of the reasons why Peter is so busy directing donor traffic into Zambia is because his office is largely responsible for drumming up the recent interest in AIDS in Africa, through its vigorous media campaigns. Peter recognises the power of public relations.

'I have a full-time team just putting out information and in the last two years, there's been a positive change in terms of global awareness of both AIDS and AIDS orphans. It snowballed with coverage in *Newsweek, Boston Globe, Village Voice, New York Times, Herald Tribune* and *Washington Post.* Between September and December in 1999, we hosted nine television crews.

'I'm a great believer that communication is one of the biggest assets you can have, if you can manipulate it to get your point of view across. It can liberate resources and change policies. You can use it as a sledgehammer or as a scalpel. It doesn't always work. Sometimes you get burnt when people portray it badly, but for every bad journalist, you get half a dozen good ones.

'The biggest danger when you're portraying suffering is the pornography of depiction. We have to be careful we're not promoting just another black child deserving charity. We have to portray the positives. It's easy to show yet another African failure, whereas in fact the amount of good work going on is unbelievable. The vast majority of orphans in this country are already being looked after by communities, without any external assistance.

'The solution is going to be a 20- or 30-year one so we've got to make sure that the money that comes in now, which will wane in a few years because there'll be another sexy subject, doesn't get lost. Everything that comes in must go towards creating an environment that will allow people to operate better, and not restrict them.'

The UN can help countries to organise their response to AIDS. It has money, so its representatives do get the ear of politicians, but they still have to play by the rules of the country they're operating in and be sensitive to local suspicion of interfering expatriates. It's a tricky task. But Peter and his team have managed to gain the trust of sometimes indifferent politicians, co-ordinate the other donors in the field and begin to put AIDS orphans on the international agenda. No mean feat.

'There is hope', says Peter. 'The incidence rate of HIV amongst young women is dropping and donors, UN and government know more, work together better and have agreed priorities. Donors aren't spraying money everywhere now. Maintaining the momentum when other commitments come along will be the biggest challenge. But you've got to look at the positives. We're winning … Most of the time I feel that. The story here is not the difficulties we're fighting against to get stuff done. It's remarkable how much is being done, given the circumstances', he insists. 'It's a glass half full.'

Section IV

Children Alone

9

A Mother to Her Brothers

A Child-headed Household's Story, Johannesburg, South Africa

'Our relatives don't come. They don't want to see us. I don't know why. Some of them came before my parents died. Some of them. Right now, they don't come. No one visits us. I don't know why. They live close but we don't see them. When we last saw them, it was at the funeral. That was the last time. I feel angry because … Why don't they come to visit us?'

Molatela is a gorgeous 17-year-old from Sebokeng, a township outside Johannesburg where some of the worst massacres of the apartheid era were perpetrated. She has a shy, appealing smile and she cares about her appearance. She keeps up with fashion and frequently changes her hair. She lives in a small, box-like house; one of thousands lined up along the township's dusty roads. Under the same roof are her four brothers. The oldest, Ngwako is 21, followed by Matome who is 14 and Nakampe who is nine. Pheega, the baby of the family, is three and HIV-positive.

One week in July 1999, they lost both of their parents to AIDS. The family of children is now going it alone. Under the circumstances they are not doing badly.

No relatives offered to take them in. Extended family relations were strained before their parents died and even if relatives had offered, the children would have been reluctant because it would have meant leaving the family home and being split up. They want to stick together.

Molatela has become the family's new mother. When she speaks, she repeats phrases with an air of slight bewilderment.

'My father died first and we buried him on Saturday …' She trails off and looks panicky, 'I've forgotten the date … The funeral was very big. And after we'd buried him, my mum died at 12 o'clock on the Sunday. She was so ill in hospital that they didn't tell her that my father had died. They didn't tell her. But I don't know whether she knew, because the day before my father died, I went to the hospital to see her and she told me that she'd dreamt about him. In the dream she saw that he'd died. I told her, "No, my father hasn't died." On the Tuesday, the family came to tell me that my father had died. It was winter.

'My mum was always sick. Maybe since '95. But my father was only sick since June this year and he died in July. Very quick. It was a shock. I didn't know he was sick too.

'At my mother's funeral, there were so many people. Maybe 200. There were four buses on the way to the graveyard and there were lots more at home who didn't go to the grave because there just weren't enough buses. Some of the neighbours helped me to cook for the people.'

For four years, Molatela and her brothers cared for their mother at home, and later their father too. She learnt about AIDS through caring for her mother, not from teachers or leaflets and posters. She knows nothing of taking extra care when handling blood and other bodily fluids. No one has taught her.

'I found out my mother had AIDS, one time when she was cooking and she cut herself with a knife. When her blood came out, she said, "No, don't help me." But she didn't tell me she had AIDS. I couldn't understand why she wouldn't let me help her with her blood. Another time she said, "I have AIDS." She was trying to tell me, but I thought she was joking. Finally one day, I overheard her telling her friends. They were talking together and I heard her say, "I have HIV." My brothers heard it too. After she'd told these friends, they went out crying, and I said to myself, "OK." My parents didn't actually tell us but I talked with my brothers about it. I said, "I heard them talk about AIDS. They say they have AIDS." And my brothers said they heard it too.

'I didn't know AIDS. I didn't know what it was, but when I saw them sick, I believed they had it because they got so thin. And their tongues were ... sort of ... furry and they had purple spots on their arms. They coughed a lot and were always sleeping. Sometimes, she was OK. Sometimes she was so sick she'd go to the hospital. Then she'd come back better and then she'd go to the hospital again. When she was better she was herself and we could laugh. And she would cook. She could really cook.

'I remember how I often used to go into town, shopping with my mum. And one time we went out to dinner at Nando's [a chillied chicken restaurant]. Just us, the girls. We were joking, laughing. It was a special day.

'My mother was a cleaner in somebody's house. But only for one month. After that, she was sick and my father told her to stop working. He was a mechanic. He fixed trucks. Sometimes he'd go to work in another city and stay there a month, maybe two. But he'd always come back to us.

'I have a good memory of 31 December last year. We were at home. We were listening to music and my father was dancing to jazz. We were laughing. Everyone was dancing and laughing.'

The children's home is secure. The parents had paid off the bond before they died. They have running water, a flushing toilet, a stereo, television and fridge. They have enough space. Most importantly, the house contains memories of their parents, some happy, some painful.

'Sometimes it seemed like when my mum was better, Pheega was sick. When he was better, she was sick. All the time, there was sickness.

'I looked after my parents until they died. My big brother helped with my father. He washed him and I washed my mother. No one else helped us … They didn't come. I don't know why.

'Before they died, my mum told her friends about having AIDS. Some of them were frightened and didn't come to our house again. I didn't tell anyone about what was going on at home because some people, when they knew that my mum was dying of AIDS, they looked at me like … I don't know what. So I didn't tell. I knew that's how they would act.

'But I did tell my best friend, Precious. When I told her, she understood because she'd helped me when my mother and father were always at home. She'd seen. She knew it was AIDS but she wasn't frightened.

'When they saw my mother was ill, some of the neighbours brought food. But some of them didn't come because they knew it was AIDS. They just didn't come any more. And some of them didn't come to the funeral. Even now, the neighbours don't speak to us. I tell myself if someone doesn't talk to me, there's nothing I can do to force her to talk to me. Some of them make me cry. Yes, they make me cry. Why won't they talk to us? Why won't they say, "Good morning"?'

After a month of struggling in isolation, Molatela and her brothers were informally 'adopted' by Gail Johnson, who runs Nkosi's Haven, a residential home for destitute, HIV-positive women and their children in Berea, a crowded, crumbling district in central Johannesburg.

Gail is flamboyant. She has bright, hennaed hair, big eye lashes and long pink nails. She lives at running pace, with one hand on the steering wheel and the other pressing a mobile phone to an ear. She sweeps into a room, constantly having 'one of those days' and greets everyone with a theatrical, 'Hello darling.' She jokes, swears and laughs heartily. She is also warm and fearless of emotional involvement with exceptionally needy babies and children. As well as two grown-up children of her own and an adopted, ten-year-old, HIV-positive son, Nkosi, Gail's home is also a registered place of safety for abused and abandoned children. The Child Protection Unit sometimes delivers them to her in the middle of the night. They are hers for anything up to six weeks. Sometimes longer.

Gail shows her emotions. On one occasion she is confronted with Mary, a 20-year-old woman, who arrives at her door with a baby she gave birth to the day before. She wants to abandon it and the hospital suggested she try Gail. A depressed-looking, older woman-friend accompanies her and holds the baby. Both women are unemployed and homeless. Mary's boyfriend has kicked her out because the baby is not his. She is adamant that she does not want this baby. She wants him looked after by a 'proper mother'. The older woman confirms Mary's determination to give the child up. She wants someone to take the baby before Mary abandons it in the street.

Both women look dejected as they eat food given to them. Mary's eyes search the faces of the people in the room, imploring them to understand and help her out. She does not seem to want to explore other options. It slowly emerges that she wants to return to her boyfriend. She cannot do that with the baby. She seems helpless and unhappy but she has made up her mind.

Gail fluctuates between caring and toughness. Again and again, she checks that Mary understands the implications of her decision and its permanence. Finally, Gail agrees to take the baby. She makes Mary promise to get herself to family planning every three months for a contraceptive injection until she is married and ready for children.

When it is time for Mary to leave, she says goodbye to her baby. Named 'Gift' on his birth certificate, he is so new that his umbilical cord is still clipped with a peg. She cries. Gail cries, hugging the woman and asking if there is anything that can be done to keep them together. There is nothing to be done, and the women leave in sadness. Gail is bereft. She keeps repeating, 'She gave away her baby.'

It was a monumental decision to witness. The child lay, uncom-prehending, in the midst of this maelstrom of emotion. Gail takes the little bundle home. Later, a detective from the Child Protection Unit visits with the necessary paperwork. He re-names the baby 'Tulani' (Quiet One). The next day, staff from Johannesburg Child Welfare Society turn up to take him away. Gail cannot understand why they have decided to place him in an institution to await adoption, rather than risk his bonding with her. She does not always agree with agency decisions.

Gail probably annoys some people because she is a bossy, outspoken white woman with scant regard for political correctness. But she gets things done. She has made a huge difference to the quality of life of one family of AIDS orphans in Sebokeng. She calls them 'my babies'. Once a week, she and the project's social worker, Mosibudi, drive out to see them with an abundance of food, clothes and concern.

Without the kindness of strangers, the family of orphans was heading for disaster.

'Before Gail gave us food, we didn't have food,' says Molatela. 'Sometimes we didn't even have mealie meal [maize]. Then we'd have to borrow from the neighbours that day. Some would give me sugar. Some just said, "No." If they say they don't have sugar, there's nothing I can do. My father stopped working in June when he got sick. June, July, August, we had to ask neighbours for food. Sometimes we were hungry. Sometimes we'd go to sleep without eating because we didn't have money to buy food.

'At that time, I didn't know what to do. I talked to my big brother. I said, "What can we do? We don't have food." And he said to me, "There's nothing we can do. Our relatives haven't come, and haven't given us money, so there's nothing we can do. We must just stay in the house." He had no ideas. I didn't have ideas. So we just stayed together.

'We didn't want to go and live with relatives. My grandmother on my mother's side is dead and before my father died he told me about his mother. He said that she wanted to give him something that when you eat it you can die. They didn't get on because he didn't give her money. I told my big brother that she might poison us too. So we didn't want to live with her. When she visited us occasionally, like at the funeral, we were very scared.'

Now Gail is there. She is a compassionate adult on the periphery of their lives. She gets Molatela to make lists of things they need. One visit there were brand-new school shoes and trousers for all of them. Molatela tried on her trousers. She is a voluptuous girl but the size she requested was vast. The grey school trousers hung off her. She looked embarrassed and mumbled that she would take them in. Matome tried on his shiny, unscuffed new shoes. He looked very pleased with them. The younger boys tucked into a tray of fruit.

Another week, Gail delivered towels, soap and some cooked chickens donated by a hotel that usually supplies schools but had forgotten that it was the school holidays.

One of their first lists requested ice-cream. They are optimistic children. It takes Gail over an hour to reach them in her hot little car. Another week, at the bottom of their list of necessities, in tiny apologetic writing, was a plea for sweets and *simbas* (crisps).

Initially, Gail took them food from the cupboards of Nkosi's Haven. A little later, she persuaded the children to do an interview with a local paper. Their story made the front page. 'Orphaned by AIDS, five youngsters fight off the harsh realities of life', it announced. Readers sent donations. One of the children's relatives angrily asked Gail why she had sought publicity. Gail replied, 'They were hungry.' The woman was silent. The Welfare Department is not keen to hand out money when no adult lives with them. Gail has applied for a grant to be processed through Nkosi's Haven. In the meantime, her intervention is an *ad hoc* response to their desperate situation. It is not an operation that could be scaled up. Even from a distance, it is labour intensive and expensive looking after just this one family of orphans.

Seven years ago, Gail became Nkosi's foster mother. When his mother died of AIDS, Gail took him to the funeral in rural KwaZulu-Natal. He is HIV-positive but, having only been seriously ill once and having Gail to fight for his reinstatement in a school, which initially rejected him, he manages to lead a relatively normal life. He has, however, become the world's best-known child with HIV/AIDS since he made a speech at the International AIDS Conference in Durban in 2000 and urged people not to be afraid of people like him.

He is an extraordinarily charming and confident child. Every visitor to his home gets offered tea or coffee and polite conversation until his busy mother returns. He confides that Gail is tired and he wishes he could learn to cook so that he could help her more. He knows how lucky he is.

On one occasion, Gail takes Nkosi to visit the orphans. They need to see a healthy boy with HIV. On a previous visit, Nakampe had been weeping with anxiety that Pheega would die soon, like both his parents. Gail is proud to show off Nkosi's long, HIV-positive life. He survives, without the benefit of expensive anti-retroviral drugs, on a regime of good nutrition and lots of love and care. She talks openly about AIDS, illness and sex in front of Nkosi. She explains why she wants the orphans to see him. Nkosi is obliging. He is more worried that his face, which is painted like a dog after a school art class, will smudge.

Mosibudi joins the crowded car on this expedition. As well as counselling the residents at Nkosi's Haven, she also works at a hospital's AIDS clinic. She is unhappy because she has seen two of her patients die that day. They had been with her since 1994 and she has supported them through HIV to full-blown AIDS and now death. She is depressed and tetchy. 'Don't ask me why I got involved with Gail, this Mother Theresa', she snaps.

But as the journey goes on, she relaxes and after an hour of banter with Gail she is a different woman. In the back seat, Nkosi grins at their rude jokes. Gail will not make the trip to Sebokeng on her own. She only feels safe going there accompanied by a black colleague.

Being able to speak South Sotho, the children's first language, Mosibudi takes charge. She instructs Gail not to unload any of the food from the car until she has assessed whether any of the children's grasping relatives are around. After their parents' funeral, the children saw nothing of granny or aunts until the latter heard that there were two women coming out from Johannesburg with food. The children had to put a lock on the fridge.

'There was only half a packet of chicken in the fridge, when we got involved a month after the parents had died', says Gail, angrily. 'No housework had been done. All their clothes were dirty. The kids were neglected and depressed. This family was on the verge of collapse.'

Gail first heard about Molatela and her brothers from a local community worker, Mushathama, whom she met by chance on an aeroplane. Now she visits them every week. She hopes to find them a freezer, so that she does not have to bring food so often. But she thinks they will need emotional support and advice for quite some time. Now that Gail is involved, Mushathama has virtually disappeared from the scene.

The children are not fools. Molatela has observed adult duplicity at close range. 'My mother's sister came round to help with the ironing one day because she knew that Gail was coming. The rest of the time she didn't come.'

When Nkosi is brought to visit, Molatela has prepared some food for him. Gail is embarrassed that her son is gobbling up the orphans' supplies. Mosibudi tells her that it is good that guests accept hospitality from them. It shows that at least some people are not worried about food being contaminated or catching HIV from their cutlery.

Molatela's relief at Gail's appearance in their lives is palpable. Suddenly there is an adult in the picture who cares enough to insist that they find a phone and get in touch when problems crop up. Gail was a stranger but she wanted to know them. She is also willing to help take care of Pheega, which lightens Molatela's burden.

Pheega gets chicken pox. Every inch of his little body is covered in angry, itchy spots. He wails with misery and makes Molatela stroke his back. He does not want to be removed from his siblings and taken home with Gail. Last time he was sick, he spent a fortnight at Gail's house being nursed back to health from a serious infection caused by a perforated eardrum. But he returned to his siblings much stronger. He also picked up some English while he was staying with her because she made him say 'please' and 'thank you'.

Gail, an experienced foster mother, does not put up with misbehaviour, regardless of whether the child has HIV or not. And this child, whose mother was sick throughout his life, has not known discipline. Molatela admits that he gets his own way. No one said 'no' to him, until he met Gail. He is a stubborn little thing. At first, he refused to eat and threw food and tantrums. He did not appreciate Gail telling him off. Gail thinks he is spoilt and needs to be socialised. She also loves him. He lets Gail hug him but his resistance to going with her again is clear.

His condition is worrying. Gail is horrified that no one told her when he fell ill. He has been feverish and spotty for three days. The problem is that, even though she wants to, she cannot take him at the moment because she cannot risk him infecting Nkosi in her home or any of the residents at Nkosi's Haven. Their compromised immune systems may not be up to dealing with Pheega's vicious-looking chicken pox.

A fortnight later Pheega lies on a mattress looking wretched. Molatela has been applying ointment to his skin. It gives his face a reddish tinge. He has visibly lost weight and he has wet himself. Molatela is worried.

Gail goes to a local pharmacy and buys numerous lotions and potions. She demands that the older siblings administer them to Pheega. She warns them that she will be cross if the bottle is not half-empty at her next visit. All the fruit and vegetables she provides are partly aimed at keeping Pheega's diet balanced. She once asked Molatela what he eats. The answer was, 'Kellogg's. Three times a day.'

Molatela may not know much about what her baby brother should eat to stay healthy, but she has definitely become his mummy.

'I had to tell him that his mother and father aren't here, but he can call me his mother. He calls me Mummy. He didn't understand when they died until he saw them in the boxes. He saw them. Now he understands because he saw them in the coffins and being put in the ground. He told me, "My mum died." When he calls me Mummy, I say, "Hello. What do you want?" It's strange because he calls our big brother Ngwako, Ngwako. He doesn't call him Father.'

A month on from his battle with chicken pox, little Pheega looks a lot better. His cheeky grin has reappeared. He potters about waving at everyone. This particular crisis is over but the long-term prognosis remains bleak. Molatela amuses him, and herself, by donning a pair of comedy spectacles with a white plastic nose attached.

'Every day when we go to school, my cousin looks after Pheega. She's 24 but she's not working or going to school. She had a baby when she was a teenager so she left school. She's nice. She's not worried about looking after a child who's sick. But when he had chicken pox, I cared for him. I had to stay off school because he wanted me. He didn't want my cousin. He wanted me.'

The older children decide that, during term time, Pheega should sometimes stay at Gail's home or Nkosi's Haven. They can visit him at weekends or he can accompany Gail and Mosibudi on their weekly visits to Sebokeng. He will not like this arrangement. However, if childcare arrangements with their cousin fail or he gets very ill, it will keep Molatela in school and keep Pheega as healthy and well-fed as possible.

From a distance, Ngwako might be mistaken for being quite tough. Close up, like Molatela, he has a beguiling 'please like me' smile. At 21, he is the man of the family. Matome and Nakampe are still confused little boys. They are angry and argumentative one minute and tearful the next. They are all burdened beyond their years, but Molatela and Ngwako carry the largest load. They are still enrolled in school, but they often miss classes. Ngwako is only in his ninth year of education. In South Africa, classes include pupils of widely varied ages, because many missed years during the struggle against apartheid or have had to repeat years. It is not uncommon for people in their twenties to be studying beside teenagers. Ngwako struggles academically. It is unlikely that he will be out of school and looking for work for some time. Molatela has only one more year till she graduates, but family trauma makes it hard for her to concentrate on her studies.

'Before my parents died, when we were going to school there was no one to look after them. I was worried. At the end, my big brother didn't go to school. He told them that our parents were very sick, so he couldn't be in school. He stayed at home one week. Just one week. But the next week, when he went to school, they said they wanted to keep him out. I don't know why. They gave no reason. He's found another school to take him now.

'The thing I like most about my big brother is that he hasn't gone off with his friends. He is always at home with the family. Sometimes at the weekend he goes with his friends and they say, "Don't look after your sister and your younger brothers." But he tells them, "No."

'I worry about my younger brothers at the moment, because they don't want to go to school. I don't know why. When I talk to them, they say, "We don't do anything at school. It's boring. So we won't go." I talk to Ngwako about it and he says they must go to school the next day. In the morning they put on their uniform, but when I go to school, they don't go. When I come home at lunch, I ask them, "Did you go to school?" They say, "No." They're very naughty. When I talk to them, they don't listen to me. They listen to big brother and he tries to be strict with them. I don't know why they don't listen to me.

'Sometimes, when I talk to them, they hit me and I must run away. They hurt me, sometimes. If I ask them, "Can you wash your clothes today or do something else to help me?" they hit me because they don't want to do chores. Then I scream at them loudly and it makes them want to beat me more, so I have to run away. They listen to Ngwako. He and I are always talking with each other. We watch television together and we eat together. But it's me who must prepare food for them.

'Before my mum and my dad died, they didn't teach me about cooking or washing clothes or cleaning. Right now, I think of how things have changed. I knew I must cook and do the cleaning and other things like this, so I taught myself. No one told me how. It was very hard to learn to cook because I didn't know anything about it. Sometimes my brothers help me. Other times they don't want to. When I ask them, they say, "I'm going to my friend's", or "I'm too busy."

'Although, I'm cooking, washing, cleaning till late, I never feel like leaving my family. When I'm not at school, I stay at home. I don't have time to go out. And I don't want my friends to visit me. Only my best friend, Precious, comes here. I don't want the others to visit me because after my mother and father died, some of them made themselves at home in our house, cooking and eating, without respect. Before my parents died, they'd come and just sit. They wouldn't make themselves so at home. It annoys me they behave differently.

'I don't know any other families like us. I talked to Precious about AIDS and she doesn't know anyone else like us either. But recently, my uncle (the one whose daughter looks after Pheega) told my grandmother (the one with the poison) that he has a … I don't know what … on his private parts. He told my grandmother it was like he was having AIDS. That sign. He said he saw that sign on my father. But he does not know for sure that he has AIDS. He just saw this sign of AIDS or STDs [sexually transmitted diseases] on his private parts. Are they different things? Anyway, he's worrying about it. But he doesn't go and get the test. I think he is scared.

'Precious has been my friend for years. She comes to help me. When I'm worried about something, I talk to her about it and she comes to me. But, with some problems I first go to Ngwako. After

I tell him, we decide whether to talk to Gail or Mushathama, our community worker. Like when we got the big electricity bill. It was R670 [about £67]. On Wednesday they switched off the lights at 12 o'clock and they wanted the money. I didn't go back to school. I talked to my big brother and then I went to Mushathama. It was a long way on the bus. Then I went with her to the office and she paid it. And we got light again on Thursday.'

As well as love Molatela probably, sometimes, feels anger and resentment for her dead parents and needy siblings, but she does not admit it. She admits only the melancholy and resignation she feels. She frequently struggles to find the words to describe her experiences, but she does not cry.

Despite the trauma of losing her parents and the risk of losing her baby brother, Molatela seems remarkably resilient. Even as she holds the present together, she manages to look forward.

'When I finish school next year, I'm thinking of becoming a sound engineer in the music industry. I don't have any idea how but I think my subjects are right. I like science and technical drawing. My big brother doesn't know what he wants to do.'

Since their basic needs have been taken care of, the improvement in this family's circumstances is dramatic. The first time Gail visited, the house was filthy and the children despairing. Within a month, some laughter has returned and the house has been cleaned up. Hand-washed clothes hang on the line in the yard. They have come a long way in a short time.

Molatela beams when Gail arrives at their door. Gail tells her she looks lovely and jokes that, perhaps, next time she will bring condoms with the fruit and vegetables because there will be boyfriends queuing up at the door. Actually, Gail fears for Molatela when word gets out that there is an attractive, lonely and vulnerable orphan living there. She has talked to her about condoms and has told her brothers that they need to protect her but they have their own troubles. Gail and Mosibudi dash in and out with supplies and hugs but do not always have time to stop and listen to the children. Gail always asks how they are doing and whether they've had any trouble from neighbours or relatives. 'No, no, we're fine', they reply almost in unison. They are still shy with

Gail. She hugs them and kisses them and they respond gladly, but do not initiate physical affection.

Molatela has had her childhood interrupted. She is an extraordinary teenager. Having nursed her parents through terminal illness, she has become a substitute mother for her siblings. She is doing the best she can to wash, cook and clean for a family of five, keep herself and her rebellious younger brothers in school, keep an HIV-positive three-year-old well, while dealing with her own grief at the loss of her parents. With food parcels and weekly visits from caring outsiders, the family is coping, more or less.

They have not so much been abused by the adult world, as neglected by it. The stigma surrounding their parents' death and Pheega's HIV status has kept people away. They remain vulnerable.

'If I knew other people like us and they needed advice, I'd tell them that they must look after themselves. They must be independent and make sure they go to school every day and always eat. Maybe if there's a big brother or sister, they must look after their younger brothers and sisters. And I would say to the big brother or sister, you mustn't take the advice of your friends because friends don't care for the family group ... I'm thinking of Ngwako's friends ... And maybe, if they are lucky like us, they can find someone who can help them ... like Gail.'

10
Falling Through the Net

A Street Child's Story, Lusaka, Zambia

A group of Zambian street kids found a stray puppy and brought it back to the shelter where they slept. It was a sweet dog. Everyone loved it. But it got sick and two days later, it died. By then, it had bitten several of the kids. But the vet refused to do a post-mortem on the puppy to establish whether it had rabies or not because of an outstanding bill of $3.

How many kids were at risk? Some volunteered to be taken to the doctor because they thought it would mean biscuits and an outing in a car. Others held back, waiting to see what happened to the first batch of volunteers. Meanwhile, a few had drifted back to the streets. The staff at the shelter called a meeting. They didn't want to alarm the kids but they had to tell them they could die if they didn't get shots. Thirty-four kids aged from 9 to 14 were identified who'd been bitten on their bare feet and hands while petting the puppy.

They were taken to a clinic. The doctor was away having lunch. There was no one around. The kids had heard that you turn into a dog before you die of rabies, so when one started barking, the rest followed suit. Suddenly, the waiting room was filled with the deafening roar of children doing dog impersonations. Eventually someone came along and told them to shut up.

Rabies treatment costs 2000 kwacha (about 40 pence) a shot. Staff scraped together the money for 170 doses, but the clinic had trouble finding enough vaccine in the whole of Lusaka, the country's capital. Staff at the Fountain of Hope shelter won't know, for another two months, whether any of their charges are going to die excruciating deaths. But they've done all they can.

Street children live close to the edge. They find it hard to keep clean, healthy or clothed. Many people despise and distrust them, kick them and shout at them. The drugs and alcohol they use to make life bearable make them more vulnerable. Shelters such as Fountain of Hope have a tough job coping with the emergencies, let alone reintegrating street-hardened children into ordinary families and schools. Some are beyond help. Glue-sniffing has irreparably

144

damaged their brain or they've stumbled into the path of a car. Too many have been allowed to fall through the net.

Fountain of Hope was started in 1996. That year, a United Nations Children's Fund (UNICEF) report estimated that there were about 75,000 street children in Zambia, up from 35,000 in 1991. People who work with the kids laugh at such estimates. Street children are too nomadic, and too frightened of authority, for anyone to count them.

By September 1999, Fountain of Hope accommodated 70 children. Six months later they had 250 sleeping there and were serving over 500 meals a day. Five hundred children are enrolled in their school.

Rodgers Mwewa is in charge. He's a flamboyant man, dressed from head to toe in orange. He drives a four-by-four around downtown Lusaka, hooting at people he knows, music blaring. When he arrives at the shelter, small boys crowd around him, pawing the car and yelling, 'More volume, more volume.'

Entering the shelter in Kamwala compound, a residential area in southwestern Lusaka, shocks the senses. The heat and squalor are overwhelming. In the big, sprawling, semi-derelict building, which used to be a bus station, kids swing on the metal bars behind which customers used to queue for tickets. The noise is like a riot and the smell of urine overpowering.

'We may reach 2000 children one day', says Rodgers nonchalantly. 'It's possible. But we don't want to just keep bringing children into the centre. It should be a transit home for children who will be returned to their families.

'When children come to us, we try to find out where they're coming from. While doing that, we give them shelter, food, and education. The first time you have contact with a child on the street, he's going to cheat you. He'll give you all the lines till you come to know him well. It's a slow process to win their trust.

'There are kids who don't want to come to the centre because there are no rules on the streets and they can make at least 500–1000 kwacha [about 10–20 pence] a day. Sometimes they're given 500 just for watching a car. It's hard to pick up those who've been on the streets for a long time.'

There are two categories of street children: children *on* the street and children *of* the street. The former work there but go home to relatives at the end of the day. They've got shelter, but most of them don't go to school. The latter are homeless and have no one to look after them. In Lusaka, these children are easily identifiable at night, sleeping around fires, in the shadows. They're the minority, but the ones most in need of help. UNICEF's research in 1996 estimated that 7 per cent of Zambian street children were actually homeless and about 40 per cent of Zambian street children had lost both parents. In Lusaka, as many as 70 per cent are now double orphans.

Capital cities have always been a magnet for street children. The metropolis is the best place to hustle for money to survive. What's new is the sheer numbers.

> 'AIDS has caused the big increase of kids coming into Lusaka since 1996', says Rodgers. 'Every day we see three to five new kids coming in, some as young as seven.
>
> 'In Africa, and in Zambia in particular, there used not to be any orphans. I mean that. When mothers or fathers died, the community elders would say to the relatives, "Who, from your family, should take care of these children?" And they'd pick someone, probably an uncle. He'd say, "OK, fine", and he'd tell the child, "I'm your father now so I'll be responsible for your school fees and your upbringing." It was solid. There was no arguing and there was nothing like what's happening on the streets now. Today, we're breaking away from that family stuff, because if a child's given to his uncle, it won't be long before he dies. They'll start looking for another person to take care of the child and that person will also die. HIV is destroying families and family bonds.'

Most street children do not know how their parents died, or are in denial. Even in a quiet moment, few will acknowledge that their parents died of AIDS.

> 'When we talk to them about HIV,' says Rodgers, 'most of them will tell you, "My mother died. My father died. That's why I'm on the streets." But they say their dad died of meningitis, tuberculosis or diarrhoea.' Rodgers sighs. 'Some of their parents died quite early on when HIV was something no one wanted to talk about. But now, people are talking about it more freely ... although not really in public, like at funerals.'

Many street children die young. Cut off from mainstream society, they rarely get the education that might protect them from AIDS.

They are far more at risk of rape than children with homes to sleep in and they tend to start having sex at a vulnerably young age. Even if they know about HIV, safe sex is not high on their list of priorities when, for some, sex buys food.

> 'On the streets, children are engaging in homosexuality, and most of them have sexually transmitted diseases which increase the risk of HIV', says Rodgers. 'When it gets bad, we take them all to be checked at the clinic and those that are infected get treated.'

He doesn't know how many children are HIV-positive. Testing is too expensive and there doesn't seem much point because little could be done to help the children even if they knew their status. HIV isn't the only health hazard on the street. Many children have got malaria at the shelter and about once a month, a child is killed or maimed in a car accident. The streets are a violent place to live. Children get scarred in fights – the burning sticks that keep them warm at night also make fearsome weapons. The public's sympathy for orphans swiftly dries up when they become fierce little street brawlers.

'We've tried to tell everybody that these children don't like being on the streets, but they still get trouble from the police and the public', says Rodgers.

Emmanuel, a shy, religious man and one of the project's founders, comments,

> 'The kids really fear the police. They used to get beaten for loitering at night. There's now a policeman who talks to them about the law. They do know the rules but when you're on the street, there's a lot of freedom and they learn harmful behaviour off older people. They're also used for petty crime. The legal implications come later when they get caught by the police who take them to the cells, where they're mixed up with adults. Then we go and bail them out.'

Fountain of Hope is not the only organisation concerned about street children in Zambia, but it is the only one with volunteers out on the streets every night. The others are more like orphanages. 'It's not easy, always to be on the streets with those children', says Rodgers. 'Some staff leave, but the strong stay. This year, we linked up with Project Concern International [PCI], which is funded by the American government. They keep us going. They're really encouraging.'

Rodgers is grappling with a computer package in PCI's offices in a leafier part of Lusaka. As the project has expanded, he's been forced to become more businesslike. Staff of street kids' projects are not always the most diligent administrators. Paperwork seems dull and unimportant when there are kids knifing each other outside. PCI is helping Rodgers to write funding proposals. Emmanuel writes thank-you letters to donors.

One day some jet-lagged Americans arrive bearing plastic bags of second-hand clothes and shoes from their church. They're on a mission to see whether this project deserves more support. One lady asks primly how many cents in a donated dollar are spent on the kids and how much on staff salaries. Barby Rasmussen, an American employee of PCI, knows where these visitors are coming from. She patiently explains that Fountain of Hope's staff are all volunteers, but that they receive a stipend and that PCI is trying to raise money for proper salaries for them. She gently prods Rodgers into telling these potential donors the story of how he set up Fountain of Hope. They're impressed. He's only 28, but seems older (except when he's mock-punching people and asking boyishly, 'Are you a fighter?'). He arranges for them to hear the kids singing (but probably not the kids' favourite song, 'Fight child labour with an AK-47'). The visitors are charmed.

Foreign money has paid for new premises for the shelter, but they need more money to finish it. Five minutes' walk from the original shelter, the new one is bigger, more modern and has enough space for a game of football. Fifteen girls already live there. The boys, if unwatched, join them.

Rodgers says that the shelter gets *muzungu* (white) visitors every day and the kids have come to believe that whites have the money to make things happen. So they're quick to ask visitors what they've brought for them. When it's clear that gifts aren't forthcoming, they dissolve away. A few say they're off to beg at traffic lights and laugh at one of their friends – a slightly aggressive boy who's been insistent that a visitor should buy him shoes – for being drunk. They try to shock. They're keen to tell visitors that they all smoke *dagga* (marijuana), 'Except him', and they point at an undersized six-year-old, who limps and looks like he doesn't really know where he is. They ask a visitor from Johannesburg if street children there sniff Bostik (glue) and whether they suffer too. In Lusaka, the kids who don't make enough money to buy glue, sometimes sniff *jenkem* instead – fermented human sewage, scraped from pipes and stored in plastic bags for a week or so, until it gives off numbing, intoxicating fumes.

At the shelter, Rodgers looks like a king; resplendent in his orange outfit with brocade at wrist and ankle. Perched on the only bench outside, he eats lunch and orders kids to fetch fizzy drinks for visitors and staff. Skinny kids sit on the ground with their *nshima* (sticky maize paste) and vegetables.

A child comes up to show Rodgers his finger. It's swollen and a strange colour because one of his friends bit him. Another child is hobbling about with an open cut on his foot. Few have shoes. All are filthy.

They wear an eccentric assortment of donated clothes. One boy dons a feminine, purple, woollen jacket over his naked torso. Another wanders about looking slightly sinister in a homemade gas mask. It's a split bottle tied tightly around his head. Kids kick a football made of tightly packed plastic bags.

There are rules at the shelter, but enforcing them is a battle. At night, over 200 kids sleep on mats. Three staff patrol, trying to minimise sexual activity between kids and break up fights that erupt when boys keep each other awake.

'When you're dealing with street kids,' says Rodgers, 'You have to take time to talk to them every now and then. Each of our street educators is in charge of about eight children and they report on the progress of each child. Twice a week, we hold meetings with all the children, when they tell us their problems and what they think we should do about them. For instance, they told me, "We're angry with that member of staff. We're going to stone him." It could be something big or something trivial, but either way, you say, "OK, let's talk about it." All that stuff. You have to identify a problem, and go in immediately.

'Whenever we throw a street kid out of the centre, we give him reasons. There was one child who was very violent, and big and muscular. He was very influential. Every kid was afraid of him. So I'd talk to him every now and then. I wanted to use him to bring other street kids into the centre. He became a very good peer educator because he was able to convince other kids that the centre was a good thing and they'd listen. I trusted that guy so much I started giving him more responsibilities, like being in charge of food. And he was happy. But then he started abusing his power. He'd say, "The children should eat beans today." And the staff would ask, "Why?" and he'd say, "Because I say so." He was trying to undermine them, and it became a problem.

'And he'd take it upon himself to beat up the boys for not closing the gates. I'd ask, "Why are you doing this?" and he'd give me excuses, but do it again. We'd talk to his friends, and they said, "Ya, he does this and that ..." So we asked them, "What should we do about it?" And they said, "Chase him out the centre." So we told him, "The children have decided you shouldn't be here."'

Rodgers now pays the 20-year-old's rent for a place nearby and has sent him to mechanics' school. 'It's a problem when the kids get older and you have to find them something to do. We've seen about five into jobs.'

Most of the children are in their early teens. Fountain of Hope has started its own 'community school' for them. During the morning, there are six different classes going on in the noisy heat, under the corrugated sheet roof. Crumbling concrete walls vaguely separate them. Some rooms have a few benches, but others just have a pile of rocks for furniture. One tiny classroom has so many children squeezed into it that it's hard to spot the teacher.

Classes are interrupted for visitors. The kids rise and chant, 'Good morning, visitors.' They're being taught maths, English and science by a group of volunteers but it's hard to imagine anyone being able to concentrate on anything amid the hubbub. Maybe ten to 15 kids will graduate from four years of this 'community school' and be able to attend a proper government school. For the rest, this is better than no education.

John, who wears a polka dot skirt across one shoulder like a cape, says he's 16 but looks twelve. He proudly shows off his exercise book in which he has painstakingly copied a teacher's instructions: 'Clean the house', 'Wash your hands before eating', and 'Eat healthy foods'. He wants to be a driver.

'There's only one boy who's a problem right now,' says Rodgers, 'because he wants to go to formal government school. We'll try and get donors to support him. He's becoming a problem. He *really* wants to go to school.'

Rodgers is talking about Abraham, a serious-looking 17-year-old who frowns a lot. Even though it's hot, he wears incongruously formal trousers and a grubby navy jacket over a light yellow shirt.

He stands out in the crowd because he's more smartly dressed, speaks more English and is bigger than most.

'I come from Ndola [a copper-mining town in the north]', he says. 'My father died six years ago. I was 14 and living with my mum and three brothers and four sisters. One time, I came home from school and asked my mum for money for shoes and books. She gave it to me, but I lost it. I spent it on beer. On my way home, I met my big brother. He's eleven years older than me and my family's first born. I was too scared to go home because he was looking at me funny and asking me about the money.

'So from that time, I ran to the streets, just a few miles from my family. The guys who were there taught me how to find money, like parking cars and begging and stealing.

'I didn't make much money. Not enough to go back home. Just enough to buy food and beer. It was so difficult, but I managed. Not a good life. You don't sleep well. Bad food. And by then, I was fighting with the police. I was fighting all the time. Sometimes drunk. Sometimes beaten by the police or other people. Something like that.

'It takes time to get used to the streets. You go through stages. First, you get to know a few people and make friends, but you can't win any fights so you're just one of the young ones. The next stage is your friends knowing you well, but there are others; some you beat, others beat you. Then there's a stage when you can beat them all or do more of something than they can do. It's that stage you reach by my age.'

Abraham gets into his stride telling how he rose through the ranks of street children.

'I've managed to earn my level and beat other guys on the streets. You can prove yourself by, if you see another group, starting a fight with them or drinking or stealing something.

'I don't have a gang. These days, it's like, "Today I play with this person. Tomorrow I play with that one." In Ndola I played alone. It was very difficult for me to make a strong relationship with others. But at least here we are looking out for each other. It wasn't like that in Ndola. We'd help each other with favours like cigarettes, but not look after each other. But here, there are older ones who look after the young ones, and there's others who are like ...'

He trails off, unable to articulate how it feels to have people care about each other enough to do more than just extract survival favours.

'After a month in Ndola, I came here because the other kids were telling me there was plenty of money in Lusaka. You can do business. You can do everything. So that's why I came here. I thought it was going to be easy to find money, but it wasn't. I did some jobs like watching cars for their owners and then Mr Rodgers found me. When he asked me to come to the shelter, I kept saying, "No", because I was fighting for money.'

A crowd has gathered around Abraham as he tells his story. He doesn't seem to notice until one of the boys butts in and says something to him.

Abraham translates,

'He says, "*Now* I'm saying the truth." OK, it was like I was in a bad way. I was fighting for money and the way I got money ... I used to drink so that, even if I beat somebody or if the police chased me, I could run and not feel fear or the pain of a beating by the police. That's why I was always drunk. I felt lucky if I was drunk so I was drunk more times than not. That's how I lived.

'When I was on the street, I didn't understand my situation. I used to say, "I don't care, even if I die today or tomorrow, as long as I'm a human being." I kept saying, "I'll never surrender." That's where I was when Mr Rodgers picked me up. Then I began to understand a little bit. But it takes time even if somebody wants to be changed.

'In some ways, it was good on the street because I could do anything I wanted. I felt powerful and like I could beat all the people: other kids, strangers walking down the road, everyone ... If I saw someone and he passed bad comments about me like, "Ah, that one, he's a street kid", I didn't ask, "Why does he say that to me?" I'd just look up and start fighting. I was angry all the time.'

At this stage in his life, Abraham was a time bomb, primed with anger and envy.

'I was angry about everything because I'd see the rich people's things. You have money, house, clothes, security guards, everything. You are sleeping well. But me, I'm sleeping on the street. I'd be thinking, "Why are they like this? Why can't I be like them? So let me fight for what they have." That's why I was so angry most of the time. Can you understand that? That's why I was fighting. It was the only way I could find money and food ...

'When I couldn't look after cars, I'd break into Indians' shops. They're bad guys. Each time, I knew that maybe this one might kill me. When I was begging, I liked the *muzungus* because some of them would understand my problems and give from the heart, but others – blacks like me – used to swear at us and tell us, "Go to your father." So? My father's dead. I'd ask myself, "Why is it like this? Why don't those people want to understand? They want us to be bad."

'But I gradually changed. After a while, I decided, "I can go to school and achieve more than others with homes. I can be like you."'

He carries a heavy load of shame about stealing from his mother.

'She came here once, but I don't want to go back home because of what I did to her. I was a bad guy. Very bad. She's forgiven me but I haven't forgiven myself. Not yet. I'll find someone who can sponsor me to go to school, and then I'll go back and help her and make her proud of me. I want to go back to my mum, but I can't because it can't be like this. It's going to take time. Maybe I'll go back if I get sick, but I'm healthy now. I'm still fighting. Fighting all my life. But this time I'm fighting to go back to school.'

Even though Abraham is now determined to get back into a normal school, it's not that simple. Rodgers is going to try to make it happen, but Emmanuel is pessimistic. There are upper and lower age limits in Zambian state schools and Abraham's big, so it's unlikely any school would bend the rules for him.

Community schools were started to give children who'd missed starting school by the age of nine the chance to catch up by the end of the seventh grade, by cramming seven years of education into a four-year curriculum. However, few manage to transfer into formal education afterwards because they're either too poor to pay for the fees, uniform and books, or because they don't make the grade academically. Lots of community schools have opened in the last few years, offering free tuition to more children, and older children, who wouldn't otherwise get it. But quality varies. They're unregulated and teachers are usually unqualified. Initially community school kids were older than their peers in the government schools, but over time the age of kids in community schools has fallen. It has become a parallel system for poor kids. Abraham wants more than this.

'Before, when I was at school, and when I was on the streets, I wanted to be a soldier. But now I want to be a geologist. I don't know when I'll start at school. Soon. Soon. I'm fighting for that. Can you help me?'

It was romance that prompted Abraham to leave the streets.

'It took a year for me to decide to come to the shelter. When I first visited, I saw some girls who live nearby and I thought, "I like that girl. She's nice. I think I'll come again." So I cleaned up for her. I washed and got new clothes at the centre. Then I thought, "She won't like me if I go back to the street." And it's then that I decided I wanted to be like normal people. The girls' families gave me good advice. At the time I was stealing, and they told me what jail was like and how I couldn't do anything without going back to school. And I was also thinking a lot about mum. So that's why I came to the centre.

'The rules at the centre were the hardest thing. No fighting, no stealing, no drinking and no smoking. It was very hard to get used to it, but people were patient and I had one of my good friends here too. But I still drink and smoke *dagga* sometimes. The centre is better than the streets. And I enjoy playing football here. We play often. I'm good.'

The crowd agrees with him. He has their respect.

'We've made the league. We're winning', says Abraham.

Football is important in Zambia and nowhere more so than at Fountain of Hope.

In 1993, the whole Zambian national football team was killed in an aeroplane crash. Lots of children came from the Copperbelt towns to mourn in Lusaka. Rodgers estimates that at least a thousand of them became street kids. Some were stuck in the city without money for the bus back. Others merely used the disaster as a pretext to come to the capital, there being nothing for them back home.

Through football, the Fountain of Hope kids engage with the outside world, or at least a few local teams. Teams are picked on merit. There's no charity involved in this area of the project. The kids, who are talented enough to be selected, can take pride in their talent. The team fosters a sense of belonging for its members and supporters. The players are all over 17 and look less malnourished than some of the small spectators.

The boys put on their assorted kit. Most have shoes. Some have socks. Others have 'Africa against AIDS' T-shirts. A few blocks away, at the grounds, their coach has them doing vigorous exercises. The nets are the only clue that this rough ground is a football pitch. Rodgers drives across it and parks. He always supports his boys.

But the match is cancelled. The pitch has been double-booked by the school that owns it.

The following day is a public holiday. Another match is planned. Rodgers, in a tracksuit, Nike trainers and back-to-front baseball cap, looks the part of a football manager. Everyone's excited about the match. Some of the younger boys have put chalk on their faces. Some of the older ones have been drinking.

But the opponents fail to turn up.

There is palpable disappointment. Eventually, the team jogs off the pitch and they change out of their kit at the edge of the field. Suddenly there's a commotion. The next minute, Rodgers is pulling a belligerent, drunken lad off the pitch. It's Abraham. With the boy's lower arm in a vice-like grip, Rodgers, who's much taller and stronger, leads him away. A crowd of kids follows the action back to Rodgers' car.

At the shelter, Rodgers is engrossed in conversation with Abraham in the tiny staff room. Lots of other boys have crammed in to watch. Rodgers is containing the emotional emergency.

Keeping in with the teenagers is hard. The kids are volatile. Relationships are fragile. It's really hard to get them off drugs and out of trouble. They lose a lot of kids back onto the streets, especially when the dry weather comes and some kids feel they haven't got the shoes and blankets they were promised.

None of the founders could have foreseen how big their project would become. Rodgers complains that he can't find a wife because he works all the time and women don't understand why he works with 'those dirty kids'. One volunteer says that he doesn't want to miss a single day, because there would inevitably be a problem and then the kids could accuse you of not being there for them. He's trying to compensate kids who have lost trust in adults. Like so many of the staff, he's in danger of burning out.

There's so much fire-fighting at Fountain of Hope that there's little time for thinking long-term. Staff at every street children's shelter talk of trying to reunite kids with their families and training local women in business skills so they can provide for their own children and foster a few extras. But building bridges with reluctant families takes time, especially if they live in distant villages and are afraid that the child has picked up city gangster habits. Finding foster parents willing and capable of handling ex-street children is rarely possible either. The shelter is stretched just coping with the children's immediate needs – food, basic education, shelter, pills and plasters, football and trustworthy adults. And more kids keep coming to town.

Shelters for street children are necessary, but they're far from ideal. Only the most resilient children make it off the street and out of such places unscathed. A decaying building packed with 200 young men sleeping and fighting together has an unhealthy amount in common with a prison. The inmates are not forced to stay but institutional life is only marginally more gentle than that in jail. Rodgers points out the 'head boy'. Was he elected? 'No,' laughs Rodgers, 'he fought for the title'. Street children don't have much choice. They have to keep fighting.

Conclusion

AIDS makes Africa's future seem bleak. Life for many Africans is already poor, unhealthy and short; AIDS is making it tougher still. Over the next 20 to 30 years, the virus will make life poorer, sicker and shorter.

No one knows what the psychological impact of the epidemic will be when almost every family has lost someone to the disease. Survivors will not be able to shake off the effects like a dog coming out of water. All around them teachers, nurses, businessfolk, civil servants and relatives will be growing ill and dying. Life will be full of delays, cancellations and funerals. As health economist Alan Whiteside suggests, 'In the absence of strong leadership, there will be feelings of panic, dislocation and disaffection.'[1]

Adversity can make people strong, but it will be an unusual AIDS orphan who gains anything from the epidemic. The damage from growing up alone will be deep and, in some cases, permanent.

AIDS will hurt children in a number of ways. Child mortality will increase, as will levels of malnutrition, illiteracy and child abuse. The number of children living on the street, fighting in wars, committing violent crime, joining gangs and abusing drugs and alcohol will rise.

More children will die, if not in their early years from HIV, then perhaps from neglect after their mothers' deaths. Because many people believe that all children born to HIV-positive mothers will inevitably be infected too, many babies will be abandoned. Relatives sometimes wrongly assume that an orphan is going to die and so don't spend money on medicines for treatable childhood illnesses. A motherless child often has no one to ensure that she receives her inoculations. Street children are more likely to die young.

AIDS sets off a vicious spiral. As adults die, families grow poorer. As families grow poorer, children go hungry. When children are hungry, they grow weak and vulnerable to infectious diseases. If they have inherited HIV from their mothers, this leaves them more vulnerable still. Many grow up with stunted bodies and minds.

More children will drop out of school to care for dying parents, earn a living, do household chores or raise younger siblings. Missing out on school will make them less employable. It may also leave them ignorant about sex, AIDS and condoms.

The prospect of so many unhealthy and unhappy adolescents is frightening. Peter McDermott of UNICEF-Zambia is concerned that

'We will have a generation of illiterate kids whose only formative experience has been one of sickness, death and marginalisation. We're not talking about individual children. We're talking about a group mentality, and their own nurturing ability in the future as parents, if they're not seeing positive role models and being parented.'

More children will be abused, because they lack shelter and protection or because selling sex is their only means of survival. Abused children are more likely to take greater sexual risks or find themselves in abusive relationships in adulthood. The trauma of rape can destroy people's self-esteem. Orphaned girls are particularly vulnerable to sexual abuse because they've assumed adult responsibilities, such as caring for dying parents or raising siblings, without the maturity to understand quite what has happened to them. South African paediatrician Neil McKerrow observes, 'These children lose the joy of their childhood and the skills that childhood develops in children ... The girls are so susceptible to sugar daddies. They just need a little attention.'

More children will end up on the streets. Recent research in Brazil found that kids who live on the street are at risk of psychological and physical damage because of a variety of factors: parental loss, minimal social support, drug abuse and having sex younger. In 1991, 80 per cent of inmates in prisons in Sao Paulo were former street children.[2]

Crime will escalate as more children steal to survive and join gangs in search of a surrogate family. More will abuse drugs and alcohol to numb their pain. Some will suffer permanent brain damage from sniffing glue or other intoxicants.

'I fear for the future,' says John Munsanje of Children in Distress, a non-governmental organisation (NGO) in Zambia. 'because anyone who has not enjoyed love has a high chance of having a spirit of vengeance. It's subtle now, but as they grow up and start to notice the opportunities they've missed, they'll be physically able to express their dissatisfaction.' Subdued, he adds, 'I see more crime coming. More serious crime.'

Increased instability and the risk of riots by hungry, unemployed young people will make investors nervous. Already, firms are looking at the impact of AIDS on productivity when considering, for instance, whether to sink money into southern African mines. If the environment becomes too risky – too many employees dying, too many expatriate engineers killed or too much machinery stolen – they'll pull out or stay away. Unemployment, already widespread in most African countries, will get worse.

The US Central Intelligence Agency (CIA) warns, 'The severe social and economic impact of infectious diseases is likely to intensify the struggle for political power to control scarce state resources ... This will challenge democratic development and transitions and possibly contribute to humanitarian emergencies and civil conflicts.'[3] These will be harder to contain as the epidemic will also have weakened national armies and international peacekeeping forces. In Africa, soldiers have a higher HIV prevalence than civilians.

The CIA is worried that the 'lost orphaned generation' may be exploited by political groups for their own ends, for instance, as child soldiers. Children are already deployed by guerrilla factions in northern Uganda, Liberia, the Democratic Republic of Congo, Sierra Leone and several other countries. To break the morally restraining ties of community and tradition, warlords sometimes force child soldiers to take drugs or to kill their own parents. Orphans, with no such ties to break, could be even simpler to mould into adolescent killing machines.

There are even some who speculate that the current violence in Zimbabwe and Congo may have been sparked by the feeling of hopelessness afflicting a generation who know they do not have long to live. Assuming, in line with national statistics, that about a quarter of the followers of Zimbabwean President Robert Mugabe are HIV-positive may help explain the violence that erupted in the Zimbabwean countryside in 2000. If you expect to die within a decade, you have little to lose from trying violently to seize the property of those richer than you.

Africa after AIDS will be an unpredictable place. What will happen to the minds of a generation that grows up alone, poor and ashamed by the stigma of the disease that killed their parents? Some will suffer depression. Others may lash out.

A whole generation is carrying a millstone of sadness from their childhood into their adult years. Those who bottle up their grief will probably be the most susceptible to depression. Girls, especially, may turn their distress in on themselves. This will make them vulnerable to exploitation. Desperate to be loved and accepted, they may be less assertive in negotiating wages, choosing friends or insisting that boyfriends use condoms.

Look into the eyes of a typical orphan, and you can see a child begging for approval. Take Rose, the 21-year-old Ugandan mentioned in chapter 2, who was cast out by her relatives a decade ago. Her pain is still close to the surface. Even after all these years, the memory of being rejected by her relatives still scars her. As she talks about the experience, it is all she can do to hold back the tears.

Molatela, the 17-year-old South African from chapter 9, is similarly traumatised. Burdened with the duty of bringing up her brothers without parental support, and ostracised by her neighbours, she is old beyond her years. Orphans like these two are often too meek and sorrowful to confront those who treat them as second-class citizens because of the way their parents died.

Others may react more forcefully. Angry with their parents for contracting AIDS and leaving them stranded, angry with social workers, politicians, police and passers-by for broken promises, meanness and brutality, these children, boys especially, may come to express their grief and confusion through violence. Seventeen-year-old Abraham on the streets of Lusaka, in chapter 10, struggled to understand why rich people treated him with contempt for begging. He responded by stealing, drinking and fighting.

A few orphans will overcome all obstacles. They'll win scholarships and find good jobs. Many, especially female orphans, aspire to enter caring professions such as social work or medicine. A few, more often boys, aim to win back respect from relatives who have snubbed them by becoming rich and powerful. But the stars will be the exceptions.

The poor often take a fatalistic view of life. In Africa, where AIDS is drastically shortening lifespans, such fatalism may grow more widespread. The United Nations has calculated that in countries where 15 per cent or more of adults are infected with HIV (all of which are in Africa), at least 35 per cent of boys now aged 15 will succumb to AIDS.[4] When teenagers hear such gloomy predictions, will they lose hope? Even if the statistics don't reach their ears, they will surely observe that the funerals they attend at weekends are often of people not much older than themselves.

As street children witness their friends die, as well as their parents, they may become more blasé about life and death. Abandoned and unloved, they may take more risks with their own lives, and, in some cases, with other people's. Watching AIDS cut short lives all around them, some young Africans may decide that they might as well live fast, spend what money they have and pack lots of sex and children into the 30 or 40 years they can now expect to survive.

Having children is extremely important in Africa. With or without the threat of AIDS, most Africans will continue to have lots of them. The fear of dying young and leaving children orphaned will not be much of a deterrent. But the birth rate will fall for other reasons: HIV makes women 20 per cent less fertile, HIV-positive women will often die before their potential child-bearing years are over and some children will contract HIV from their mothers. Few of these children will survive past infancy.[5]

Life carries on, even when death is everywhere. Prominent Zambian AIDS activist, Clement Mufuzi, said,

'In the West, this would be considered antisocial [fathering children knowing that you are HIV-positive], but children are the most important thing in our lives. A man or woman without children is seen as cursed. Without children you cannot live normally. You are despised by people around you. Nobody will take away my right to have children, whether I suffer from AIDS or not. Life is already sad enough.'[6]

Despite this catalogue of anticipated horrors, the orphan generation is unlikely to reduce Africa to anarchy. The epidemic may somewhat increase the likelihood of civil war, but it is unlikely to be the catalyst to start one. Why? Because AIDS orphans have been isolated by their experiences. They're unlikely to band together and organise themselves into an angry adolescent army. Who would they fight against? A child-headed household suffers behind its closed front door. Street children are more often beaten by the police and other adults than vice versa. Unhappy and hungry orphans will probably raise crime levels in the countries where they are the most numerous, but slowly, not suddenly or dramatically.

What can be done? The most useful thing would be to slow the spread of HIV. Although there is no cure for AIDS, and unlikely to be a vaccine for several years, we do now know how to avoid contracting the virus: abstain from sex, be faithful to your partner or use condoms.

We have learnt from places like Thailand, Senegal and Uganda that governments can lead the battle against AIDS and that we are not powerless in the face of it. But in most of Africa, leaders are still uninterested or daunted into paralysis by the magnitude of the crisis.

The tasks are mammoth. Changing sexual behaviour is exceptionally difficult. Simply talking about sex is hard enough. Former South African president Nelson Mandela was a great and saintly leader, but even he failed to grasp the nettle. Once, early on in his presidency, he began to talk about AIDS in front of an audience of traditionally-minded South Africans. The audience's reaction was one of shock and disgust. They protested that talking about sex and condoms would encourage immorality among the younger generation. Mr Mandela, who was reportedly uncomfortable with the subject in the first place, barely mentioned it in public again.

Reaching children before they become sexually active, and get into habits they will be loath to break, is really the only 'window of opportunity'. Despite what many people believe, there is no evidence that sex education prompts kids to rush out and have sex. On the contrary, research suggests that it persuades young people to wait a little longer before becoming sexually active.[7]

But what of the children already orphaned? Even if the AIDS epidemic was magically halted, there would still be over 13 million orphans.

There is no simple solution. There isn't a government, NGO or 'childcare model' that alone can solve the problem of how to prop up all the over-extended families *and* catch all the children who fall through existing safety nets. The sheer number of orphans is too great. But governments, donors, NGOs and community leaders can learn to confront the crisis and try to exorcise the stigma that still surrounds AIDS. More effective planning and co-operation would follow. A willingness to innovate, and to allow others to do so, is crucial.

People often believe that the way they bring up their children is the best way, indeed, the only way. Likewise, many people who are running programmes to help AIDS orphans believe that what they're doing is the only way forward, and that everyone else, if they had any sense, would follow their example.

This is rarely true. There is no single formula that will work for all orphans. People should learn from each other, but there should always be space for individuals or organisations to experiment and see what works. Beyond setting certain minimum standards, governments should not try to dictate to NGOs how they should care for orphans. Many minds are likely to be more creative than one or two.

There is a need for shelters for street children, orphanages and people like Heather Reynolds at God's Golden Acre in chapter 5. As the number of AIDS orphans swells, all options will have to be tried. Family life is best, but where there are no potential foster parents, institutions will have to take the strain.

Given the scale of the crisis, people will have to ditch their prejudices. If the only potential home for a black child is with a white family, or vice versa, the child's immediate needs should trump the arguments of those who oppose transracial adoption. If a child needs to care for dying parents, it may sometimes be helpful to train him or her to earn a living. Anything that smacks of child labour will appal many people, but pragmatic NGO workers see this sort of thing as making the best of a bad situation. Development workers need to be realistic. The very poorest communities are unlikely to be self-reliant for a long time, and orphanages are not, always, the worst option.

Recognising that we haven't yet discovered the ideal project that could be scaled up to solve the problem, UNICEF-Zambia advocates a mass of small projects in chapter 8. Small projects have many advantages. Because of bureaucratic delays, big national projects often take years to set up; small projects are much quicker. National projects require lots of money; in countries where corruption thrives, this attracts powerful thieves. In a small local project, by contrast, the intended beneficiaries are in direct contact with the person who controls the purse strings. They will probably notice if money is being embezzled, because there will suddenly be less available for them. Being close to the grassroots, small projects are more responsive to changes in local conditions. If they grow too big, they can lose touch with the communities they're trying to reach.

Bongi Zengele and her colleagues at the Thandanani project in South Africa, featured in chapter 4, have been on a steep learning curve trying to set up community childcare committees. They have made progress, but it's been slow and hard-won. They have neither the funds nor the capacity to scale their project up to national level. But they are prepared to share the lessons they have learnt. Such information-sharing is crucial if others are to imitate their triumphs and avoid their mistakes.

Programmes need to be transparent and cost-effective. Not only to keep foreign donors happy, but in order to provide the best help possible for the largest number of children. Transparency is easier; it is simply a matter of keeping proper records. Cost-effectiveness is tougher. Should money be concentrated on a few children, as The AIDS Support Organisation (TASO) does in Uganda? By putting a few orphans through boarding school, TASO gives them the chance to become teachers or even doctors. But if the money were more thinly spread, would it give more children a better chance of survival?

The Association François-Xavier Bagnoud (FXB) tries both approaches in chapter 7. In the Luweero District in Uganda, it helps potential high-fliers by paying a few scholars' school fees. At the same time, it puts food on the table of families who have taken in lots of orphans by giving the guardian a grant to start a business. A hundred dollars for a bull, or a microloan to start a tomato-selling business, can change lives. But if assistance is diluted too much, or distributed through nebulous community structures without sufficient safeguards, it can disappear without trace.

Foreigners can help. As well as money, they can offer the kind of expertise and overview that is possible when you have the resources to commission research and fly around the continent talking to lots of people doing similar things. But there is a responsibility in giving money. Donors must have people on the ground who understand local politics. Otherwise, wasteful blunders can occur. Unwise donors can end up paying for cars and mobile phones for local politicians because they're unable to say 'No' to requests 'from the community' for fear of being deemed imperialists.

Apart from lack of money, one of the biggest obstacles to responding to the AIDS orphans crisis is the stigma that still exists around the disease in many African countries. Stigma breeds secrecy, which makes it hard to spread the message of safe sex. But stigma can be overcome. In Uganda, where everyone has friends or relatives who have died of AIDS, people are no longer labelled immoral and kicked out of their jobs and homes if they test positive for HIV. This makes it much easier for Ugandans to pluck up the courage to get tested.

The rest of Africa should consider following Uganda's example. Getting yourself tested demonstrates personal responsibility. Knowing you're infected early on gives you time to plan for your children's future. But outside Uganda, fear keeps people out of the testing clinics. It stops HIV-positive mothers from using infant formula to reduce the risk of infecting their baby. Many are terrified of the stigma of being seen *not* breast-feeding. It inhibits them from so much as visiting their child, if that child is in an institution known to be for HIV-infected children such as Beautiful Gate in chapter 6. It prevents people from insisting on condoms to protect themselves or their partners.

Confronting the stigma is something that even poor governments can do. If politicians are televised kissing HIV-positive babies and shaking hands with AIDS patients, life for AIDS orphans might grow less frightening and lonely. Villages might offer more support to the affected families in their midst, rather than shunning them in misplaced fear of contamination.

Some development workers believe the stigma is made worse by donors and NGOs who categorise AIDS orphans separately from other children in order to assist them, for instance, by paying their school fees. Mary Crewe, director of the University of Pretoria AIDS Research Unit in South Africa, argues that it is absurd to refrain from helping orphans for fear that it may inspire envy. The needs of AIDS orphans, she says, should motivate us to improve things for *all* children.[8] She argues that the state should take responsibility for AIDS orphans and build good, new institutions for them. It shouldn't be left to 'romantic notions of community' or over-stretched extended families that, in overcrowded urban situations, are more at risk of child abuse, crime and violence.

Given slender budgets and limited competence, however, governments will not find it easy to follow Ms Crewe's prescription. The increase in numbers of needy children will mean that, other things being equal, the average standard of care that the state can provide will fall.

South Africa is the only country in the region that could obviously afford to provide AZT or Nevirapine to reduce the risk of mother-to-child transmission of the virus. Providing these drugs and milk formula to all pregnant HIV-positive South Africans would, according to one academic's calculations, save 8,000 babies' lives and R800 million (about £80 million) of taxpayers' money every year, but the government refuses to go down this route.[9] No one knows why. It may be connected with president Thabo Mbeki's much-publicised doubts about whether HIV causes AIDS or his suspicion of western drug firms. He was once reported to have accused America's CIA of conspiring to make South Africa waste a fortune on American-made drugs.

A more sinister explanation was hinted at when Parks Mankahlana, the late presidential spokesman, suggested, in unguarded comments to *Science* magazine, that there was little point saving the lives of children who would grow up to be a burden on the public purse. 'A country like ours has to deal with that,' he said. 'That mother is going to die and that HIV-negative child will be an orphan. That child must be brought up. Who is going to bring the child up? It's the state, the state. That's resources you see.'[10] After the furore that followed, he denied saying these things, although the interview had been taped.

Perhaps 19 million people have died of AIDS around the world. At least another 34 million may die of it over the next decade. HIV prevalence appears to have peaked among some groups; teenage girls in Zambia, for instance. But most AIDS deaths come years after HIV prevalence starts to decline. And in some countries, such as South Africa, prevalence is still rising.

Could anything positive come out of this disaster? It is possible, but not likely. Some people predict that family and community bonds in Africa might grow stronger in the face of the epidemic. Perhaps, but the African family was tight-knit and mutually supportive before AIDS. The disease has served mainly to put it under strain. That strain will probably not destroy it, however. Blood is thick, even if invaded by a virus. Far more families are valiantly struggling to care for their orphaned members than are stealing their inheritances.

Amid the misery caused by AIDS, ordinary people are performing extraordinary acts of generosity.

In September 2000, Grace, a Zulu woman who works as a housekeeper in Johannesburg, lost her boyfriend to AIDS. When she went to his funeral in rural KwaZulu-Natal, she met his three small children, whose mother had died, probably also of AIDS, two years previously. Her late lover's mother introduced them with the words, 'Children, this is your new mother.' They immediately clung to her and wept with her.

Asked later how she felt about inheriting this responsibility, Grace replied, 'It's OK. I promised him that I would take care of his children. So I will.'

Notes

Preface

1. UNAIDS/WHO epidemiological fact sheet on Zambia (UNAIDS, June 1998).
2. Hunter, S. & Williamson, J., *Children on the Brink*, 2nd edn (USAID, 2000), p. 16.
3. Pisani, E., Schwartländer, B., Cherney, S. & Winter, A, *Report on the Global HIV/AIDS Epidemic* (UNAIDS, June 2000), p. 7
4. 'Buddying' was the term given to the befriending-someone-with HIV/AIDS arrangement started by volunteer gay men in the US in the 1980s.
5. Whiteside, A. & Sunter, C., *AIDS: The Challenge for South Africa* (Cape Town: Human & Rousseau and Tafelberg, 2000), p. 70 and personal communication with Dr Neil McKerrow, Grey's Hospital, Pietermaritzburg, South Africa, 13 November 2000.
6. Levine, C., 'The new orphans and grieving in the time of AIDS', in O'Dane, B. & Levine, C. (eds), *AIDS and the New Orphans: Coping with death* (Westport: Auburn House, 1994), p. 4.

Introduction

1. Personal communication with Dr Tony Johnston, Population Communication Africa, Nairobi, Kenya, 18 December 1999.
2. Pisani, E., Schwartländer, B., Cherney, S. & Winter, A., *Report on the Global HIV/AIDS Epidemic* (UNAIDS, June 2000), pp. 5–7.
3. loveLife, *The Impending Catastrophe* (Johannesburg: Abt Associates South Africa Inc, 2000).
4. Hunter, S. & Williamson, J., *Children on the Brink*, 2nd edn (USAID, 2000).
5. Hooper, E., *The River: A journey to the source of HIV and AIDS* (London: Little, Brown, 1999).
6. Cooper, W., *Behold a Pale Horse* (Light Technology Publishing: Flagstaff, Arizona, USA, 1991).
7. *Time*, 11 September 2000.
8. Marais, H., *To the Edge: AIDS Review 2000* (University of Pretoria, 2000), p. 55.
9. Pisani et al, *Report on the Global HIV/AIDS Epidemic*, pp. 43–53.
10. Pisani, E., 'The Naked Truth', unpublished commentary (June 2000).
11. South African *Mail & Guardian*, 31 March 2000.
12. Gilgen, D., Campbell, C., Williams, B., Taljaard, D. & MacPhail, C., *The Natural History of HIV/AIDS in South Africa: A biomedical and social survey* (Johannesburg: Council for Scientific and Industrial Research, 2000), pp. 70–1.

13. Pisani et al, *Report on the Global HIV/AIDS Epidemic*, pp. 19–20.
14. Stanecki, K., 'The AIDS Pandemic in the 21st Century: The demographic impact in developing countries' (US Bureau of the Census). Paper presented at the XIII International AIDS Conference, Durban, South Africa, 9–14 July 2000.
15. Quattek, K. & Fourie, T., *Economic Impact of AIDS in South Africa: A dark cloud on the horizon* (Johannesburg: ING Barings, April, 2000), p. 8.
16. South African *Business Day*, 18 April 2000.
17. Pisani et al, *Report on the Global HIV/AIDS Epidemic*, p. 8.
18. *The State of the World's Children 2000* (UNICEF, 2000), p. 103.
19. Schönteich, M., 'Age and AIDS: South Africa's crime bomb?' *African Security Review*, Vol. 8 No. 4 (1999), p. 34.
20. South African *Sunday Independent*, 13 June 1999.

Conclusion

1. Whiteside, A., 'AIDS Demography', *AIDS Analysis Africa* Vol. 11 no. 2 August/September 2000, p. 3.
2. Campos, R. et al. (1994) 'Social networks and daily activities of street youth in Belo Horizonet, Brazil', *Child Development* 45: pp. 319–30 quoted in Feuerstein, M., *Poverty & Health* (London: Macmillan, 1997), p. 56.
3. Noah, D. & Fidas, G., 'The global infectious disease threat and its implications for the United States', (CIA, January 2000), pp. 5–6.
4. Pisani, E., Schwartländer, B., Cherney, S. & Winter, A., *Report on the Global HIV/AIDS Epidemic* (UNAIDS, June 2000), p. 23.
5. UNAIDS, *AIDS Epidemic Update* (December 1999), p. 17.
6. Van Kesteren, G. & Van Amerongen, A., *Mwendanjangula! AIDS in Zambia* (Amsterdam: Mets en Schilt, 2000), p. 11.
7. Pisani et al, *Report on the Global HIV/AIDS Epidemic*, p. 40.
8. Crewe, M., 'Others will not save us.' Paper presented at the HIV/AIDS orphans workshop: Building an urban response to protect Africa's future, Johannesburg, 21 July 2000.
9. Skordis, J., University of Cape Town, quoted in South African *Mail* and *Guardian*, 21 July 2000.
10. *Science*, 23 June 2000.

List of Organisations Featured in this Book

Any of the following would be grateful for donations.

Introduction

Catharine Watson, Editorial Director
Straight Talk Foundation
PO Box 22366, Kampala, Uganda
www.swiftuganda.com/~strtalk
Tel: +256-41-543 025
Fax: +256-41-543 858
Strtalk@imul.com or strtalk@swiftuganda.com
Bank account: Stanbic Bank Uganda Limited (A member of the Standard Bank Group of South Africa), Kampala, Uganda, Account no: 0140060560304. Name: Straight Talk

1 Mbuya's Story

John Munsanje, Manager
Family Health Trust
Children in Distress (CINDI) Project
P/B E243, Makishi Road, Lusaka, Zambia
Tel: +260-1-223 589
Fax: +260-1-222 834
Fht@zamnet.zm
London bank account: Barclays Bank Plc, Knightsbridge, International Banking Centre Dept, PO Box 391, London SW1X 7NT, UK Sort code: 20-47-42. Account no: 60603058. Name: Family Health Trust

2 Extended Families

Sophia Mukasa-Monico, Director
The AIDS Support Organisation (TASO)
PO Box 10443, Kampala, Uganda
Tel: +256-41-567 637
Fax: +256-41-566 704
tasodata@imul.com
TASO dollar bank account: Barclays Bank Uganda Limited, Kampala Road, P.O. Box 7101, Kampala, Uganda. Account no: 4024987

Beatrice Were, Co-ordinator
National Community of Women Living with HIV/AIDS (NACWOLA)
PO Box 4485, Kampala, Uganda
Tel/fax: +256-41-269 694
nacwola@infocom.co.ug

Pelucy Ntambirweki, Executive Director
Uganda Women's Effort to Save Orphans (UWESO)
PO Box 8419, Kampala, Uganda
www.uweso.org
Tel: +256-41-532 394/5
Fax: +256-41-532 396
uweso@imul.com
Please contact them to discuss the safest way to send donations.

3 Strangers Step In

Ros Halkett, National Programme Manager: HIV/AIDS
South African National Council for Child & Family Welfare
PO Box 30990, Braamfontein 2017, Johannesburg, Gauteng, South Africa
Tel: +27-11-339 5741
Fax: +27-11-339 8123
cwo@icon.co.za
Charity no: 000-834
South African bank account: ABSA, Eloff Street, Johannesburg
Branch code: 50-29-05. Cheque account no: 01241010291

4 Childcare by Committee

Linda Aadnesgaard, Director
Thandanani Association
PostNet Suite #30, Private Bag X9005, Pietermaritzburg 3200, KwaZulu-Natal, South Africa
www.thandanani.org.za
Tel: +27-33-345 1857
Fax: +27-33-345 1863
thandanani@alpha.futurenet.co.za
Charity no: 006-136 NPO
South Africa bank account: Standard Bank, Longmarket Street, Pietermaritzburg
Branch code: 05-75-25. Current account no: 052131327. Name: Thandanani Association

5 Hope in the Hills

Heather Reynolds, Director
God's Golden Acre
PO Box 331, Cato Ridge 3680, KwaZulu-Natal, South Africa
www.togan.co.za/gga
Tel: +27-31-782 1417 or 782 3337
Fax: +27-31-782 3337
gga@wandata.com

Yvonne Spain, Co-ordinator
Children in Distress (CINDI)
PO Box 1659, Pietermaritzburg 3200, KwaZulu-Natal, South Africa
www.togan.co.za/cindi
Tel: +27-83-467 7124
Fax: +27-33-345 1583
yspain@sai.co.za
South Africa bank account: First National Bank (Main), Pietermaritzburg
Branch code: 22-08-25. Account no: 50950394780 Name: Pietermaritzburg
& District Community Chest (Charity no: 002-14 NPO). Please specify that
the donation is for CINDI, and the Community Chest will ensure that they
receive it.

6 Institutionalised

Toby Brouwer, Director
Beautiful Gate Ministry
PO Box 263, Muizenberg 7950, Cape Town, Western Cape, South Africa
www.beautifulgate.org.za
Tel: +27-21-371 7107
Fax: +27-21-374 8237
Bgate.crossroads@iname.com
Charity no: 005-086 NPO
South African bank account: Standard Bank – Blue Route
Branch code: 02-56-09. Account no: 072029773

Liz Taylor, Fundraising Secretary – AIDS Children
Nazareth House
PO Box 12116, Mill Street 8010, Cape Town, Western Cape, South Africa
Tel: +27-21-461 1635
Fax: +27-21-465 6414
nazhouse@netactive.co.za
Charity no: 002-958 NPO
South African bank account: Standard Bank, Adderley Street
Branch code: 02-00-09. Account no: 070215936. Name: Nazareth House
UK bank account: Barclays Bank Plc, Hammersmith Group

Sort code: 20-35-90. Account no: 90989878. Name: Nazareth House AIDS Fund. Please put your contact details in the reference block so they know where the donation came from.

7 A Hundred Dollars for a Bull

Anil Purohit, Interim Executive Director
The François-Xavier Bagnoud US Foundation (FXB)
651 Huntington Avenue, Boston, Ma 02115, USA
www.orphans.fxb.org
Tel: +1-617-432 3511
Fax: +1-617-432 3578
afxbanilpurohit@hotmail.com

8 Foreign Aid or Interference?

Laura Boardman, Donor Development Manager
United Kingdom Committee for UNICEF
Africa House
London WC2B 6NB, UK
www.unicef.org
Tel: +44-207-405 5592
Fax: +44-207-405 2332
Lboardman@unicef.org.uk

Lisa Szarkowski, Director, Media Relations
U.S. Fund for UNICEF
333 E. 38th Street, 6th Floor
New York, NY 10016
USA
www.unicefusa.org
Tel: +1-212-922 2643 or 1-800-FOR-KIDS
lszarkowski@unicefusa.org
Please make cheques payable to 'U.S. Fund for UNICEF'.

9 A Mother to her Brothers

Gail Johnson, Director
Nkosi's Haven
PO Box 403, Melville 2109, Johannesburg, Gauteng, South Africa
Tel: +27-11-726 7581
Fax: +27-11-726 4852
Nkosishaven@worldonline.co.za
Charity no: 008-995 NPO
South African bank account: Standard Bank, Melville, Johannesburg
Branch code: 00-61-05. Account no: 401024881. Name: Nkosi's Haven

10 Falling through the Net

Rodgers Mwewa, Executive Director
Fountain of Hope Association (FOHA)
PO Box 32320, Lusaka, Zambia
Tel: +260-1-265 191
Fax: +260-1-261 181
rodgersmwewa@hotmail.com

Others

The United States Agency for International Development (USAID) has produced some useful publications about children affected by AIDS that can be found at:
www.usaid.gov/pop_health/dcofwvf/dcwvprogs.html
and www.synergyaids.com/children.htm
For more information please contact these relevant departments:
1. The Displaced Children and Orphans Fund
2. The HIV/AIDS Division
3. The Africa Bureau
The United States Agency for International Development (USAID)
Office of Health and Nutrition
300 Pennsylvannia Avenue, N.W.
Washington D.C. 20523
USA
www.usaid.gov
Tel: +1-202-712 0000

Index